Counseling Bipolar Disorder

Learning to Live

I0462135

By Terri Kovalcik

Counseling Bipolar Disorder; Learning To Live

ISBN-13: 978 1500519506

ISBN-10: 1500519502

Table of Contents

Acknowledgement; is it Bipolar Doom?

For years we "run" around being the typical bipolar disordered person who is chemically imbalanced while our friends watch and stay blissfully ignorant that there's unevenness. One day something happens and you and your friend aren't friends and it's been years since you have interacted. They don't know you anymore as you have evolved for the better of for the worse. They don't know but then again they don't know of your condition. When you meet again and you've acknowledged the condition and accepted the normalcy of it as well as every embarrassing moment, bad behavior, less than desirable actions that occurred during your life time except this time they are afraid because you told them what you have.

It is in our acknowledgement that demise occurs as perception twists its way in regardless of whether or not it's accurate. It is also in our acknowledgement of our capacity that it is our demise. As a person with a type of Bipolar Disorder who has acknowledged not only my condition but my capacity. I find it difficult to find the help without somebody looking at me with judgement not understanding that it takes a great amount of effort to discuss what is needed and in the end it's like you're crazy for admitting that you are needing help.

It is the demise of the condition because nobody can see it. It's not a visual thing. It's a behavioral condition, a mental thought pattern that only awareness of ones' self could one say the exactness of issues, anxieties, triggers, sensitivities and again it is to the demise of the self that has acknowledged.

In the "career" world most people who are chemically imbalanced due to the physical or emotionally traumatic events that broke the chemical balance can't work because the world is too much even when blissful. We try to work with the intention of wanting forever but usually the employment is terminated within a three to six month period.

The true career for persons who have the mental illness DNA where the chemical imbalance is now in full swing is in the artistic world. This extends from one end of the creative spectrum to the most intellectual of stimulus of Sciences, Architecture, and Math. Paintings, singing, dancing, acting, writing, sculpting, are just a few of the extraordinary talents that lay "untapped" as the depressive waves wash upon the brain.

Society has forgotten that even the most highly regarded people had the mental illness DNA and they had a chemical imbalance. This is what makes them forward thinkers, and the envelope pushers. If you think about it, if it wasn't for Winston Churchill do you think history would have been the same as it is now? No it wouldn't. Our past would be different because if he was in the present at the beginning of his career and he acknowledged his condition, the world wouldn't be so adept to listing to his voice, and his thoughts. They would chalk him up to being crazy. Among the "crazy" to be considered are the founding fathers of the United States and why the Constitution was created; they were forward thinkers, they wanted to create change and make the United States what they would consider the best place on Earth to live. They saw in that chemically imbalanced thought pattern that there was something amiss in the equality of persons. They created change by being themselves and society accepted them. Would society have accepted them if they had "come out of the closet" in acknowledgement? Probably not, but then again have you ever noticed when they consume alcohol that their emotions are "more"? Probably not.

At one time persons with mental illness were put into institutions thinking that was going to solve the problem but the reality is that even today we are not treated as equals. Back then they considered this thought pattern to be a disease and even today some are saying it is a disease. Society loves its movies and they are immersed in the realness of the actors and the emotions portrayed. The reality is that our actors have the mental illness DNA and are chemically imbalanced yet they are loved for this. During their career they come to realize the levels of emotions that they have is because of this condition then they come out of the closet and the world has empathy for them and they are still loved for it. Yet would be they be loved and have empathy extended if they had before launching their career.... Probably not because even today very few "normal" people understand the condition and how if emotionally coddled the person with mental illness can   flourish.

And So It Begins

Like the evolution of animals, I too evolve into what is needed to become. I'm taking the Counseling Skills Diploma Program with ICS Learn. Yes it is correspondence but it's not that easy. They have very "trixy" like questions and so you pour over the information that you scour it some more. The other positive, if you're like me, is that you can work on it all day long with having to leave your place or be at the school for a certain time period. I am goal orientated and when it comes to something I love to do, I'm all over it getting it done. The course suggests "out letting" the information so it becomes more absorbed so here we are learning to be better persons with counseling like behaviors. I will receive my accreditation and begin creating the program for my book The Bipolar Workshop.

The communication process has four essential elements: the message the sender, the channel, and the receiver creating what is called a Communication Feedback Loop.

Listening to what others say is an important part of the communication process but you must observe the body language, and facial expressions in order to be effective.

When somebody is trying to problem solve there are two ways of getting them to "absorb" what they are meaning. One way is to repeat it back to them verbatim or you can paraphrase by using different words without changing the meaning.

When somebody has their arms crossed we typically think they are angry or cross but it can also be that you are self-conscious about your person or you are comforting yourself or quite possible be cold and trying to warm up. So no jumping to conclusions. Lol.

When we are dealing with co-workers we need to exercise our patience, tact, courtesy, and show some empathy they can't help themselves, they aren't working on bettering themselves in order to cope with the daily routines our lives are made up of. So forgive them, help them, and teach them through positive action.

Everybody has a defense mechanism and it becomes quite apparent when encountering negativity and the rise of angering emotions. Some push it out of the conscious mind into the unconscious which is called repression while displacement is the transference to another, seemingly easier target.

Projection is one's own ideas, feelings, or attitudes are attributed to someone else and rationalization is justifying your actions for "logical" reasons, without really examining the true motives of behavior. There is a difference between rationalization and intellectualization which is reasoning is used to avoid the truth.

Sublimation is an instinctual desire or impulse is diverted into a socially acceptable activity. Temporary withdrawal is finding a way is finding ways to avoid dealing with painful or difficult situation.

Malingering is pretending to be sick in order to avoid dealing with an anxious situation. Of course denial is failing to accept and deal with traumatic, stressful situation by refusing to admit or acknowledge that the situation even exists. Sometimes regression happens which is returning to an earlier mental or behavioral level during times of stress.

Counseling Bipolar Disorder

Goffmans' Rituals of Interaction

Erving Goffman brought a fresh approach to the study of everyday life according to the Leonard Broom and Philip Selznick in Essential of Sociology. Two themes are central in Goffmans' work. One of them was the fate of the self in the course of interaction; meaning the way somebody is put at risk in encounters with others or how he/she manages those risks. The second them is the fate of the micro-order; that is, the many devices that are used, often unconsciously, to sustain the continuity of social life at the level of human interaction.

The Episodic Nature of the Micro-Order

The micro-order may be conceived of as made up of millions of minute and transient episodes of social life. Even where people have long-standing relationships over many years, the actual time they are in communication consists of relatively brief encounters and occasions. In this sense "society" is not an abstraction- it is made of very specific activities and communications, many of which are fleeting and precarious. To some degree, society as it is really lived in continuously coming into being and passing out of existence.

"A sociology of occasions is here advocated. Social organization is the central theme, but what is organized is the co-mingling of persons and the temporary inter-action-al enterprises that can arise from them. A normalization is stabilized structure is at issue, a 'social gathering' but this is a shifting entity, necessarily evanescent, created by arrivals and killed by departures."

Social interaction is much like theatre. There is an expressive, dramatized element designed to project a definition of reality as much as to carry out practical tasks. Shakespeare's metaphor "all the world's a stage" can be developed into a dramaturgical model of the micro-order, showing how everyday life is pervaded by features of a theatrical performance. Thus, many social establishments are divided into "front-stage" and "backstage" regions. In the front stage areas are the living room, food counters, or an idealized display of decorum and cleanliness is affected whenever outsiders are present; back stage, in the bedrooms and kitchens, performers can relax in guarded secrecy. Social performances are often staged by teams, such as the husband and wife hosting a dinner party or the doctor and nurse showing the spotless clinical efficiency in the presence of patients.

Different Kinds of Neurotic Reactions

Anxiety Reaction: The anxiety reaction is characterized by chronic apprehension. The individual often feels that something terrible is going to happen, but he doesn't know what it is as if a black cloud of fear and worry floats constantly over his head.

Hysterical Neurosis: There are two kinds of hysterical neurosis: conversion type and dissociative type. In the conversion type, the individual converts anxiety into a bodily symptom such as blindness, deafness, or paralysis.

In the dissociative type, the person may manifest such symptoms as amnesia or multiple personalities.

Phobic Reaction: A phobic reaction is an irrational fear that the individual is characterized by a constant preoccupation with certain ideas. They may be preoccupied with the idea of death, loss of status, or loss of sexual ability. The individual finds partial relief from the anxiety associated with his obsessions by performing person rituals designed to magically counteract the nagging ideas.

Depressive Neurosis: The phrase chronic dejection aptly describes the individual suffering from a depressive neurosis. He has the "blahs", is discouraged and demoralized and life barely seems worth living.

Neurasthenic Reaction: Involves feeling of fatigue, lack of energy, and general weakness. The individual feels unable to cope with his problems. The complaints of weakness have little or no physical basis.

Hypochondriacally Reaction: Is characterized by excessive worry over physical health. The individual jumps to conclusions. A skin blemish may produce an instant self-diagnosis of skin cancer, a pain in the chest is said to be a heart attack, and so forth.

Social Perception and Cognition

Although Kelly proposed that each person has his or her own set of personal constructs, a set of bipolar adjective (e.g) honest-dishonest or friendly-unfriendly" which becomes the essential terms for characterizing people. Even within common culture or subgroup, construct systems are unique to individuals. Thus, in the case of "good old Charlie", one person may interpret his behavior as friendly-unfriendly, while another person may view it as sincere-insincere, warm-cold, or outgoing-shy.

When we have a positive bias which is when impressions of people are much more likely to be positive than negative. While the negativity effect means that our impressions of people are strongly influenced by negative persons with one negative trait, regardless of whether the person has other positive, ostensibly or extreme traits and behaviors.

Implicit personality theories are a set of unstated assumptions about certain types of people or about people in general. Many people seem to assume that persons described as intelligent also tend to be friendly and not self-centered. In 1964 Wrightsman came up with that there are philosophies of human nature which means that we vary from each other in how we conceive people along the following lines:

1. The extent in which we believe people are trustworthy or untrustworthy
2. The extent in which we believe people are rational and can control their destinies
3. The extent to which people seem to be altruistic or selfish
4. The extent to which people are seen as independent or conformists

5. The extent to which we see different people as unique or similar to each other
6. The extent to which we believe that people are basically complicate and different or rather easy to understand.

We are not aware of these assumptions which influences how we form impressions and react to people. Biases and assumptions tend to persist even in the face of contradictory evidence.

Perceiving People and Things

We need to remember that there is a difference between objects and people and how we perceive them. Objects are constant over time other than usual wear and tear of time. People change over time and their characteristics often vary with different circumstances. Thus our perceptions of people can be over generalized and obsolete. When we perceive other people, they may also be perceiving us. Thus we are concerned both with forming impressions of others and rating impressions of ourselves.

People do things for reasons, to achieve their own purpose; that is, people are casual agents- we are concerned with why others act as they do. While objects like cars do not act intentionally or are being stubborn when it doesn't want to start. One of the ways that people act intentionally is to change their appearance or actions when they are aware that others are watching them. Objects of course don't change while they're being watched.

People are very complex and there is inevitably that much about them is a private, or hidden from view. Even among experts it is much easier for an auto mechanic to understand any car than a psycho-therapist to understand a person.

Categorical Thinking

We tend to form impressions and make judgements about people quite rapidly. We don't simply absorb information and apply logic but we are active in processing information, often in biased ways. Despite our tendencies to take "cognitive shortcuts", not waiting for all the evidence yet we seem to carry on effectively in our daily lives.

Every person is unique, there are no two people exactly alike yet we tend to organize our view of the world in terms of categories. People are generally categorized in terms of easily observable characteristics. We usually assign people to categories of sex, racial groups, or age. We use other observable cues such as type of clothing, speech characteristics or language, or place of work to assign people to ethnic group category, nationality or occupation.

Now a prototype are representations; mental images are typical examples. If you were to see an unfamiliar animal in a zoo, you would decide whether it was a mammal by comparing it with say a cat. You might even have a prototype of the elderly, perhaps a grandparent, as the smiling, silver-haired wrinkled, kindly person often shown on television. The extent to which a particular person resembles the prototype, and the extent to which you allow for variations, will determine how readily the person is identified with the category. This information is processed more rapidly and included more frequently in the subjects' impression of the person when it was consistent with the prototype.

A stereotype refers to a particular kind of prototype for which "a consensus exists among members of a group regarding the attributes of another". They are conceived as fundamentally negative, motivated by prejudice and enabling us to assume that members of a disadvantaged out-group and are "all the points to numerous examples of which exist without basis in fact.

It's important to understand that stereotypes enable us to organize our thoughts about people, reducing complexity to manageable proportions where we might otherwise interpret the behavior of people from other groups. While the content of the stereotype may or may not be accurate, its existence aides our capacity to makes sense of the world.

In 1983 Kruglanski concerned himself with "freezing", which happens when the person refuses to consider other possible explanations for a situation, or new evidence which is not consistent with the person's conclusions. In the end people become closed-minded under certain circumstances. One of these is when we feel a high need of structure, a sense of certainty under pressure, such as "little time" then we tend to reduce confusion and come to a decision quickly. Another condition related to "freezing" is a   fear   of   being   wrong.

Mental Health Changes for Persons with Bipolar Disorder

It is in the opinion of this author and person with a type of Bipolar Disorder that services that do not exist should exist.

Residential Care Aids for mental illness patients who have children. Parent who have children and have Bipolar Disorder have a difficult time being the 24 hour parent. They need some help, I can't say how much or how little. It really depends on the person and it doesn't matter if they are married or single, regardless of income.

Residential Care Aids for mental illness patients who are episodic in nature; during these times of depression and helping to maintain an evenness. If a client can't make it in to an appointment for counseling then the counselor goes to the client. Also regardless of income or marital status.

Now these Residential Care Aids will need some training in mental illness and this is where The Bipolar Workshop comes in handy because it is a reference tool. You're also supposed to write down what you learned in that chapter; embedding it into your memory.

A new Disability Tax Credit Certificate designed Specifically for Person with Mental Illness. The current form is not good enough. This tax credit certificate should be designed for those who are episodic in nature; they work usually three to six months then employment is terminated by either them or the employer. Also the persons who have worked but no longer able to function in a workplace setting for periods of time should have a disability tax credit certificate as well. There should also be a list of typical symptoms, you can use my books as a reference and a bunch more on the internet.

Every workplace needs to use The Bipolar Workshop as the New Mental Health Handbooks so the repeated exposure is stopped in the workplace. I don't work anymore and sometimes I want to work but hem I'm overcome in anxiety due to repeated exposure. This book is critical in the Customer Service Industry due to the customers that are shopping in stores; let's prevent repeated exposure.

If I didn't tell you about the things that need to be changed how would you know? It's not like others who have what I have realize or publicly acknowledge their condition and still want to make the world a better place even living in 93% Social Isolation due to the world and how it is.

Just wondering, what are you doing to make this world a better   place?

Mental Illness and Criminal Acts

With the latest escapades of the mental illness that is running rampant and of course the all the expression of dismay and some haven't made it through the last mass murder and I'm having a hard time dealing with everyone's dismay and one understands why so I'm going to enlighten all of you.

It all started at the beginning of time when the original body was born the mental illness DNA. This person went through life experiencing all kinds of things. There were good things and there were bad things. The bad things affected this individual which set forth a break in the chemical balancing in the brain. Each time this person had a repeated exposure situation; something that occurs more than three weeks creates anxieties and every time that same issue comes up it makes the condition worse.

If we think about life and how traumatic this world can be one person can have at least five either emotional or physically traumatic events during their life time. Unless treated to correct the chemical imbalance because as the condition worsens the person changes and is always changing, some evolving and some digressing. I can say that due to my mother's condition she no longer has the ability to re-enter certain lives. I'm not sure if she's working on correcting the imbalance but I am working on mine.

So now that we've established increasing of emotional range when a child is born from the chemically imbalanced person that is now the "balance" in that child's brain so now whenever that child has a traumatic experience their levels are worse which explains the running rampant of what has been going on for centuries, I'd say the beginning of time but then you would be scared.

I know I am because it's almost like the world is chemically imbalanced and they don't know it. With blissful ignorance gone are you glad I advised of the personal   research?

Where Does It Come From?

Maybe a better question is why is it that we consciously and subconsciously devalue ourselves many times throughout a day?

Is it the perception that we must be humble, or modest when accomplishments occur?

If we look deep beneath the surface of the fragility of the human emotional need we may find that just maybe you've been told no too often or maybe you are told you're a braggart or you've heard that you're just inflating your ego.

Whatever the case may be think about why they are saying these negative things to you. Is it because they wish they had the skills to help themselves feel better? Feeling better doesn't really take much if you think about it because it's a thought pattern process. When we go from, "aww gee thank anyone could do that" to a plain and simple "thank you" there's a change. Can you believe the difference in words and how you can feel just by accepting praise?

Oh yes accepting praise can be difficult if one isn't used to hearing it but in order to grow as individuals and get over this self-depreciation of ourselves we have to start being more positive.

Some favorite demeaning sentences are "it was all my fault", "I am useless", "this is going to be a disaster". When we do these things we are downgrading achievement, personalising faults, generalizing faults and exaggerating them.

Positive thinking is not blind optimism, it is a way to change by emphasising the positive. When you say "it went very well", "not pressing the red button was my mistake", "I am not skilled at that particular task", "the potential results of this are both god and bad. The good are _____ and the bad are _____." When we say these politically correct sentences we are accepting achievement, accepting responsibilities for certain errors, specifying areas of competence, and assessing outcomes fairly.

The Mobius Strip

At times, should we be so lucky to encounter an opportunity that is like a Mobius strip. What is a Mobius strip you ask? It is when you have a piece of paper and you wrap it around touching the other end, then drawing a line on that paper.

In life we often encounter these Mobius strips and not know it, not understanding it, become excited, up, down and all around. The level of emotion upon encountering is never the same. It is never the same because people who have a type of Bipolar Disorder are usually evolving in personality, character traits, anxieties, repeated exposure fear, past time opportunities that have potential to create a better "ness" or a complete dissolve until the next Mobius strip comes along.

Often times we find that death is among us, occurring and we turn to our family, children, aunts, uncles, cousins, brothers, sisters, grandparents, in laws, and some of those "outlaws" you call family forming a connection of way might consider a "shelter".

It's like saying, "This is my shelter; these are my people who support me, they love me, we are trying to be together." Too often when together "ness" is discovered from years of tragedy we hear the same old people saying the same old thing. In order for the Mobius strip encounter to be successful one must not listen to the admonisher's jestering of jackalitis.

When awareness comes to the table it is often to best to write down the touchy topics, the need to talk about topics, things that could be said, and how to move forward. When we write down the touchy topics it's like the first round of talking; all the emotion comes out as we write our feelings down. The second round is to a "safe" person who listens, thereby lessening the sensitivity to the topic. When the encounters does happen usually what is heard is more happy times because after all, the topic has been talked about, let go of, and being able to deal in a more "level of emotion".

Remember to take each day at a time, don't get too excited, be calm, and think of things to look forward, and think of things to look forward to; a togetherness of sharing   joy   and   love.

A Spoon Full of Sugar Helps the Medicine Go Down

Often times we find ourselves at a fork in our relationship, sometimes it's a subconscious comparative values and sometimes it's not it's more of a plea for help; "Look at me, do you hear me, do you want me, do you love me, what am I doing wrong, why do you have to ALWAYS be on that?"

During these times we need to remember that even in the darkest regions that find ourselves in these relationships we need to take a look at our part in the discourse. Are we paying attention to our partner? Often times when we tell our chosen one (could be for the moment due to comparative valuing) we miss them, they will feel wanted, loved, cared for, and empathy for their "cause" to be away.

There are times when we have to look just beyond the showing love words. Questions that we can ask ourselves are, "When was the last time we went out for dinner, or when was the last time we sat down on the couch just the two of us with no distractions; cellphones, facebook, interneting, twittering, writing and just talked or even watch a movie? Have we spent a weekend together just the two of us? Have we spent time with mutual friends or maybe over dinner?"

Quite often in relationships we find ourselves feeling alone, unloved, and not at all attractive due to the "non"ess of the partner. Take heed, you can create the change needed. When we enter into relationships we tend to try and give our best to make things work despite everything that works against the making of a healthy relationship. When we find that this relationship is not compatible we end it.

There are many times we will find ourselves wondering if the person we just met has more potential but put it out of your mind. Just because they pay attention to you does not mean they will love you the same, or that they will look after you're the same. Only your partner knows you especially after years of being together. Through thick and thin times, as the years melt into another remember the good times, the happy times you had and rekindle the love that once was there.

In the case of children being involved, here's just a reminder about what happens when parents break up; they act out, they rebel, the will challenge the new relationship partner, they will never give up hope that Mommy and Daddy will get back together, besides, just like fighting a fire; you never leave your partner behind.

We cannot turn back the clock with the last statement admonishing our part in the failure of previous relationships. We cannot want to go back to those ones because we are in a relationship and it's time to make your relationship "Fireproof" just like in the movie with Kirk Cameron; Fireproof.

Everyday can be a challenge of whether or not our perception of the relationship is working or if it is even worth the time. Just remember it is worth time, the energy, the love spent, the love incurred, the love shown helps get things back on track. We are never alone in a relationship and we all have our parts we need to be for our partner.

Relationships and Eggs

Relationships are liked cooked eggs. It may seem like a silly analogy but if you think about it, there are many kinds of relationships that a person can have just like cooking eggs.

You can have your eggs sunny side up, scrambled, basted, boiled, and poached, over easy, medium, hard, raw, as a soufflé, and as an omelette. It's really up to you how you like your eggs.

If you take this same train of thought and apply it to relationships and categorize the feelings you had in past relationships I'm sure you will find you've been having a variety of unhealthy rotten eggs served on a platter and you have been eating them up like they have been going out of style.

There are many patterns of behaviors that a person has in relationships and quite a few words about the opposite sex and it doesn't matter if you are a man or a woman, you have words to say about relationships and the observations you make about the relationships you are involved in, see in the outside world, and in the social media world.

There is no such thing as a perfect relationship. You can cook eggs to perfection and that will be as close as you get to having a perfectly good relationship that won't get angry at you, treat you like a child, berate, condone, fake, or pretending to be something else. Unfortunately eggs don't love you back especially if you're allergic to them. (haa haa)

I don't have to explain every type of behavior because the best book is Men are From Mars and Women are From Venus and from there it is like the recipe cookbook that you've been missing your whole life and wish that you'd been eating the right kind of eggs instead of the garden variety. What I can tell you is that if you want a healthy relationship (please note healthy not perfect) you must think about your values; about yourself, the things you stand for, what you are willing to put up with or endure just to have a relationship.

If you find that your relationship is a pile of rotten eggs ask yourself why, how are you perceiving this relationship, under what situational/emotional condition did you start the relationship? Ask yourself if you are a fighter; you know the one, always against everything, the polar opposite of every sentence spoken or are you the taker; always taken the verbal slander, are you the punching bag, are you being controlled in such a way that is uncomfortable for you?

Another major hurdle in relationships is how people were brought up and no single person has been brought up the same way even in family situations. Think about it, if you were the first one born you were raised probably very protectively, as a second child, the mother let loose of the reins a little bit, by the third and fourth child, well I'm sure they were coddled or just another mouth to feed. When we can forgive ourselves and our parents for all the situations that occurred from being a baby to adulthood one might be able to have a stable relationship.

Think about your and others emotional love needs, more so when you are trying to decide things as a couple. If he or she is fighting with you about something to think about whether it's worth fighting over or maybe it's just easier to roll over and play dead until the next issue arises or maybe just maybe you'll be able to arrive at a relationship that doesn't involve hurting the other emotionally.

If you're in a relationship and you keep saying it would be easier to be on your own to your relationship partner maybe you should think about what you are saying. Would it really be easier? After a while it might be because every relationship that ends is like experiencing a death. When we are hurting, slinging not so nice words and there's talk about leaving the next feelings that will be hurling towards you are sadness, fear, anxiety, and what are the options you have for extraction. Are these threatening words really necessary? Are you saying those words because you want your way and that's the only tactic you know for getting your way because if it is, you need some marriage/relationship counseling.

Every time you say negative things to your relationship you are hurting yourself and the other person and if you're doing that then maybe it's time to pack your bags and find another egg to cook. Remember negative repeated exposure kills relationships.

Internet Withdrawal Syndrome

We live in a social media world where utility, banking, "mailing system" and a new form of directory is pushing for people to use their website to rectify any issues you're having.

Everyone acknowledges the feelings of how much money all of the "land line", cellphone, and internet companies make. The emotion invoked are the typical anger, hostility when you see your bill each month knowing they make billions upon billions of dollars yet there are quite truthfully so many areas on this planet that are without the basic of necessities; running water. The use of an outhouse is a common sight in the vast wilderness.

As we slowly approach small populated areas we find yet again that internet, cellphone service greatly lacking on a variety of factors:

-not every person has the financial capacity of affording such a "luxury"

-areas of no to poor cellphone reception

-the only available "form" to these consumers is satellite.

We all know the ring a ding, ding cost with satellite, well, maybe not everyone. There is a dish fee, an installations fee, a modem rental fee in some cases and the internet plans that only allow you so much usage per day/month/can limit/slow down your interneting if they think you use it too much. A person can use a satellite internet provider where clouds affect the quality and you're stuck in a contract.

With all the cramming of "use internet" through endless tv, radio, and even website commercials one would think that is now considered as essential as indoor plumbing, heat, hydro and running water.

If this is the case why are they making billions of dollars and not filling this essential service to areas that are lacking?

I'm sure, because I've heard it before is that they are providing the latest, the greatest, "can't be without this quality of communication" to highly populated areas.

Why does that statement seem ridiculous? Is it because the highly populated areas have had these essential services for probably twenty years minimum. Over here in British Columbia as well as all over this planet once could consider us a 3rd World population as we are in some geographical areas 20 years behind in cellphone technology.

A suggestion for our billion dollar essential service providers is you could "share tower power" and start providing 2013 cellphone and internet technology to those who   don't   have   it.

The Blind Eye

In a galaxy far, far away the Rebel forces are trying to over throw the Kettle Federation. The Queen relies heavily on her minions to fulfill her proclamation to maintain status.

The Rebel Forces are led by Jedi Master Flower Boopsy....

If life were like the movies then it could be an inspiring true story or the most horrific tale of events depending on the mentality and perception of the main character.

As the main character, we are to be the center of attention, we have supporting characters that interact in the story that is being watched on a TV screen. As viewers we, as in real life while watching shows make comments that go unheard, and rightly so because it's just a TV show. When you are "tuned into" the program the music helps invoke emotion, the believability of the character and story line needs to be plausible and there are usually three things that occur before the conflict/situation is resolved. Oh the joy that all forms of entertainment can bring.

What doesn't bring joy is when we are watching TV and seeing Reality TV commercials where you end up shaking your head going, "Who comes up with these ideas any ways? Like seriously? A show about people being "smelly" that's a whole new level that screams, "We need more ideas, we can't think of any good ones." There are over six different kinds of reality TV shows and if you watch them it's a great way of identifying the signs of Bipolar Disorder. Watching what they are doing, what they are consuming, how they are reacting to things. These are teaching tools for us as we now have our eyes "Wide

Open" seeing very clearly now. This is not to say that you need to steer clear of them, it's called being aware.

If you've been watching the "show" for a while and it's nothing but repeats and now you're yelling at it then pretty soon you stop watching it because it's aggravating. This is the great thing about TV shows.

Think about it. If you could take a negative situation and push the "Off" button, hence creating a Blind Eye to the reality of what's going on wouldn't life be blissful? You wouldn't see illnesses such as cancer, paralysis, spinal injuries, and dementia. You could just go along merrily with your life whistling the Smurf song all day long.

It is an interesting argument is it not? To be asked to have a Blind Eye when it comes to the health of another person is an odd question but when it causes problems because Oppositional Defiance Disorder has replaced the blood in the veins that is supposed to keep the heart functioning what do you do? Do you keep "beating your head against the wall" or do you do something about it?

At the end of the day it all becomes too much and there is the build of one emotion; anger. One is that Jesus would not be impressed that an individual could do that to someone and more so if they care about their well-being. The other of course is that you are the evil one that doesn't care because well, they can afford to turn a blind eye.

It's a paradoxical world we live in where double standards, or as I say not as I do, and the blind eye like to roam and day   the   story   is   just   fine   for   them.

The Slapping Stand Up

With so many values, traditions, opinions, family structure, the "poor me", the "raging anger do nothing" people in life that it is no wonder that there will be no harmony on this Earth. Maybe harmony could be found on a new planet where only people who are proactive, positive, emotionally supportive, believe in excellent customer service, and in the importance of maintaining level ecosystem are allowed.

What's that? You say you'd be there and you know a few others too. I'm pretty sure that anyone and everyone who reads this will say that they belong in a colony where there are no wars, people are kind, helpful, and respectful. Yet somehow there is always one that can be found later, after of course, that is the raging anger but does nothing about it.

The frustration level that can occur when trying to help somebody like this can be like winning an Academy Award but it's the polar opposite in emotion, the similarity is the level of emotion exuded.

You're getting a slap for standing up and trying to fix the situation that they were over emotional about. In the same token you get a slap from them for not standing up for them as well. So just when you are about to take a seat you get a slap then you stand up and get a slap and it just goes on until one person changes their destructive behavioral pattern and starts appreciating or even standing up for themselves. Nobody likes somebody who complains about something but refuses to take action to resolve the situation or issue, and acts just like the rest of society who is aware but does nothing.

In this day and age we cannot afford to be single task oriented or aggressive-passive. We must have our eyes wide open because 50% of the time the person behind the counter doesn't care about their client and it doesn't have to be somebody that's working who takes advantage of you.

Being aware is kind of like playing Texas Hold'em Poker.

Putting Your Back Into It

The wave's crash onto the beach sending debris to the shoreline as it is now rid of the oceanic material that doesn't suit its needs, the same can be applied to the emotions that keep coming back. The only difference is that some are unable to be rid of the emotional debris that keeps ending up in our minds.

Once you can acknowledge, then accept that these emotions aren't healthy it is now time to decide what to do with them so that they don't keep popping back into your mind.

Reading about Bradshaw on the Family and seeing that persons who have been emotionally, physically, sexually, verbally, and or abandoned emanate the same emotional behavioral responses when "triggered". The acknowledgement of the behavioral pattern is a set-back in emotional stability. Where you once thought that you were "over this" it is in fact a lie. The acceptance of the condition typical to Bipolar Disorder to being the reason why you are the way you are the way turns out to be in fact an amplification of the qualities described which are on the most part pretty accurate when you are honest with your selves.

The rug has been pulled out from underneath you. Now what? Acceptance of these behaviors is the result of childhood traumas. When you have been able to accept the facts you have to now decide how to rid your selves that have been affected by those emotions.

Taking the example of what a "Lost Child" is, you know the one that feels like they don't belong anywhere; not in a family unit, nor with relatives, working its way through school into adult life. So here you are now, Lost Child. How is that you are going to be able to accept that you have created fantasy parent and family that have are just waiting to reconnect with you, they miss you, they love you? These words are from a fantasy image that you have created.

Yes, your Inner Child is crushed, its heart will never be the same again. Your inner child is now grieving for the loss of a fantasy not the reality. When you end a relationship with somebody it's hard to move on. You have these "missing you" feelings, "I still love you" feelings and they won't stop until there is a finality to it.

As odd as it may seem one suggestion is to have a funeral for the fantasy family. This way whenever the Inner Child starts yearning it now has a place to go and talk to the fantasy family because they are in a grave. No fancy coffin needed just a box, a pile of rocks, and two boards nailed together in the shape of a cross.

Don't be half-hearted about it because these are the parents you love more than anything in the world. Show the love in an appropriate manner; you don't need to be ordering bouquets of roses for it because that's taking it too far. If you're like me and don't have a pile of money to spend you create something to emanate the love tat you have for your fantasy family.

Don't be afraid to talk to them when you are missing them. Even though they are dead they will bring you new life as you   are   now   the   "Found   Child".

Booking Time

So here you are at home and you're waiting for your relationship partner to come home from work except he phone rings and they're saying somebody is requiring his/her services/help. Off they go, leaving you behind to do the chore at a moment's notice.

There are all kinds of emotions that come about when this happens and it feels like it's happening frequently. I can tell you that all kinds of fights can and probably do occur when something is said.

When we don't need help everything is fine but when a list starts accumulating needing your partners help and they start freaking out about doing anything for you because they work six days a week and do this kind of helping for somebody else it's time to book some appointments.

If your name is on the calendar, then there is no excuse for anyone else to take away your time with your spouse because you've written both of your names on the calendar. If you have experienced enough repeated exposure and can't take it anymore and you love this person, want to be with this person then may I suggest writing your names down over a three month period? Don't be putting your names down every day of the week because that is being selfish. Don't feel ashamed because that's what you really want to do. We have all been there but now there is a solution to save your relationship and the aggravations caused by fighting.

So grab your black marker or pen and start writing your names on the calendar as much as you feel is necessary.

Even if it is just the two of you going for a walk on your appointment it doesn't really have to be about getting work done.

A word of caution; your partner may look at you as if you are "crazy" and silly for doing this and it may not be as successful as you hope it will be but remember this; you are trying to make the relationship work. If they don't want to make the relationship work well you will see it clear as day in their reactions. Give them time to get used to this first   before   you   start   getting   upset.

The By Product of Cool

As a survivor of high school with undiagnosed Bipolar Disorder I can tell you that when you're in school you're either cool or you're not and if you're not just like I was then you were bullied.

It has been 20 years since I graduated and I can tell you that I still remember those people and I still remember what they said, how they acted. I am a by-product of their behaviors, their emotions either self-inflated or the hiding of insecurity because when it comes to anxieties it only takes a couple of weeks of constant repeated exposure and guess what your emotions have changed, you are more emotional and pretty much scarred for life if you can't move through it.

I have read lots of books and yet I am still having a tough time moving through it. There is a 20 year anniversary coming up for my graduating class and the anxiety that courses through my heart making it pound faster and faster of images of being made fun of yet again or all those people who put me down with be falsely "Oh hi, it's great to see you," then they turn around and talk about you profusely.

A prime example of that is when I went to a restaurant in my hometown and there were people I've seen before and holy doodle as soon as they left they were on their cellphone exclaiming at the sight of me.

I am Bipolar and it doesn't take a Rocket Scientist to figure when someone is on the phone and looking at you whispering quietly or someone who just had to walk by and stare with large eyes at me. I am the by-product of cool; I am 8 times more sensitive to these actions of others.

Now as much as we all jump up and down about anti-bullying it still happens even in 2103. I cannot say how bad it is, but what I can say is that if parents are anti-bullying then they should be looking at how they treat their spouses in front of their children. It is directly from The Road Less Travelled that children do as they see their parents do. So if Dad is a jerk to Mom then the child will think it's okay to treat Mom poorly. Now these actions also extend into going to school, they will act just like the parent they look up to and they will treat their peers just like how Dad treats Mom.

Let's clean up the messy house of emotional terror and maybe   the   bullying   will   lessen.

You Drive Us Crazy and We Can't Help Ourselves

Do you remember the song lyrics, "You drive me crazy and I can't help myself?" It's one of many "theme songs" that are played while persons with Bipolar Disorder are when we are trying to drive in a safe manner.

"Vrrrroooommmmmm, vrrrooommmmm let's get there now" is the typical behavior we share. Our lead foot can get us into trouble with speeding tickets as fear of being late or just wanting to be there because it seems to be taking an extended period of time while trapped in a live of five and you're going 80km/hr due to the motorhome that wants to drive at a touristy cozy 95km/hr. With no passing lane in sight the frustration builds.

They don't drive like they used to. They aren't comfortable driving the speed limit as they gather a pile of cars, trucks and logging trucks behind them. Oh sure they drive slower with their tires just over the while line unofficially saying "Pass me but I'm going to keep driving" and while they are over there it's not quite safe enough to pass. Everybody else roars by as their road rage is fully engaged. My anger boils and I begin to want to follow the person into town and take away their driver's license. *If you can't drive the speed limit and you can't pull over to a complete stop in a safe place to allow others to pass you, you should not be allowed to have a driver's license. There are Residential Care Aids available, contact your local hospital and stopping being a hazard.*

"KEEP RIGHT EXCEPT TO PASS" this is a sign people! When we are in a double lane going in the same direction and you're on the left just driving 10km/hr over the speed limit pretending you're passing the other person the Grey Poupon Mustard he asked for and we're behind you, please be aware that there is a rule that you're not supposed to do that, it is how accidents happen. Somebody suffering from other peoples' driving habits and now come across two vehicles who have been side by side for more than one kilometer; this is where I start yelling, waving my arms, and now my throat starts hurting because I've been yelling for quite some time then they finally pull over. We get through that one and then we come across somebody in the left lane doing the speed limit and the car in the right lane is ahead of the other car. The right lane car speeds up and then we start driving faster and pass both the left and right car ripping down the road as fast we can up to 130km/hr because by now we've rightly had enough. I am in control of my emotions and keep it all in my mind. Allowing me an outlet of actions I would like to do but would never do. Except maybe start taking away driver's license and honking the horn loudly at people who pull out in front of me cutting me off and when I encounter them and they can't even drive the speed limit and I show myself several times in their side view mirror indicating "THE GAS PEDAL IS ON THE RIGHT, TRY USING IT!" and sometimes I'll do the big ole' smile and wave something fierce like I'm your long lost bestest friend as I have my gas pedal to the floor trying to gather speed to pass you in a safe location.

P.S. The last part was tons of fun by the way, you should've seen the look on their faces.

"I Have Everything You Want"

I don't know about you but my heat quickens when somebody says that when I'm in the market for a newer vehicle or, "It's clean! Mint condition, has all new tires, brakes, tranny, that type of engines is the best one, it has 345 000 km (could be any number, this is just an example)" and when you go look t it, well, it's not what they said or maybe it's just that they say that about every vehicle they have on their lot.

Having Bipolar Disorder and these type of poor business conduct situations are a trigger and the emotional flow can be like a rocket being sent to the moon.

First you're in love with it, it's shiny, it has a cd player, A/C, power windows, locks, leather seats, the floor is clean no dents, some paint chips but it's SHINY!!!

You want it, oh but you dooooo want it so bad, it looks perfect and the salesman said there's nothing wrong with it. Let's just signthe paper work and go. Oh boy this is just awesome. The day couldn't get any better, as your eyes dance in delight and a smile as long as a mile is plastered across your trusting face.

You take the test drive. You start noticing things like the rug roof of the interior is falling, the brake pedal has no rubber on it, and the axles are hot when you pull over.

Second emotion enters with driven force. You are feeling betrayed. It increases as the salesperson jabbers on about what a great vehicle it is even though in your opinion it's not.

We all understand the need to make money, it's what make the world go around but do not try to pull the wool over anyone's eyes being put into the pile of negative perception that all sales persons are snakes in the grass and they'd try and sell a lemon as a bright shiny apple.

One of the hardest things in life that you will learn constantly is that there is false advertising and it is everywhere, and false marketing. For the world it's about make a fast buck. Things that once were made with pride and quality products have been replaced with cheap plastic replicas that break fairly easily. In a lot of cases nothing is what it is supposed to be. An unfortunate by product of consumerism. Society demands and somebody finds a cheaper way to make it, make it have a short life span so the consumer is continually purchasing it.

Huge sighs of relief also exit a person when they are told, "I'll do it for you. I can take this on. I need $XXXXX.XX as a deposit." Life is happening to people in every sense of the word. Whether you are the person representing or if you are the client. People seem to forget that at times in all kinds of situations all over the world. Days collide into another as each person faces the typical daily challenges. It can range from house cleaning, looking after kids, taking them here, there, pick up their prescription, drop them off here and there, go to the Post Office dealing with a relationship turmoil, while experiencing immense body pain but somehow you can get these things done. Except at the end of the day one task has been left undone; getting the paper work in. Life can be challenging and when influencers block the path it makes life more difficult.

Impatience by both parties arises but this is no time to declare it's time to take a vacation especially when you have the paper work. I've watched lawyering type movies and not once have I seen a scene where the lawyer says, "Well I'm going on vacation and if you don't do this part then I'm not representing you."

This is my perception of poor Customer Service understanding both sides of the fence. If you, the representing person, needed the paperwork that badly and knew of your clients challenges then you should've called and went to their house and things could've happened a lot faster as you are now providing Quality Customer Service.

There is a great debate about how billionaires get rich, their business conduct, and their personal life due to status but I have to say that I watched the first couple of seasons of The Apprentice with Donald Trump and with each challenge I think that I wouldn't have been eliminated and dare I say that I would've been a finalist. It is because I have a type of Bipolar Disorder that my values are like embedded mesh into my core self. It is hard for me to stand by and watch people trying to take advantage of others regardless of Mental Illness Status.

If you conduct poor business don't be surprised when your doors have been closed for you because every job (truth) requires you to adhere to the standards of The Better Business   Bureau.

Reconnection Notice for "Broken" Families

There are more than 2 million people on this planet called Earth who have a type of Bipolar Disorder and I'm going to guess that 1 out of 8 people, the family has held together. This is being optimistic. The latest statistic is 1 in 2 Canadian women have been sexually abused (which can emotionally terrorize them until death unless they talk to the "self" that is the victim).

Now one of the things about having a type of mental illness that is not known about or even considered can destroy families.

If you acknowledge that it's genetic, which means quite frankly that it is not the parents' fault. Now if you have a chemical imbalance (this is what causes those roller coaster of feelings, behaviors and of course add in Chapter 1 from The Road Less Travelled "From the Sins of the Father"; it talks about how as children we are influenced by our parents.)

From a 3rd person perspective even though it's the inner child saying that unless parents acknowledge their parents raised them, and let's get honest here: hatred, envy, jealousy, and with a fierce determination that once you left, your adult life is going to be all about you, just like one or both of your parents were.

I have learned, I have seen, I am the inner child that speaks to all the inner children of the world whose family is emotionally terrorized by the effects and affects of Bipolar

Disorder. I stand up for the inner child whose family is broken and stating, "We should be so lucky, we are still alive because what is going to happen if one of us dies without reconciliation? Are you going to be able to live in the knowledge that there comes a time to "retire" our unhealthy behaviors and "try on some new shoes?"

Besides you might find these more comfy and less emotionally terrorized by your family being "broken".

One more thing about the reconnection of families; if you are the one of the parents who wants their child back and feel like you can't because of the spouse, you need to stand up for yourself and do what your heart longs for.

What is the worst thing that could possibly happen? They want a divorce? That in itself is a very childish behavior.

Don't wait until the inner child slams the door and says, "I will not allow myself to think that I am worthy of a family."

Coming Face to Face with Reality

It's never easy to say that we are dependent upon another person or to say that we tend to find certain kinds of people, certain kinds of relationships especially when it feels so shameful and more so when you have Bipolar Disorder.

The self of self is destroyed. There is numbness in feelings; not knowing how to feel about anything at any particular time.

We delight ourselves in child-like awareness because life is better in awareness versus reality. We tend to find ourselves in abusive relationships typically when a child has grown up in a family where sexual/physical and or emotional abuse has occurred.

I was reading Bradshaw On: The Family that was written back in 1988 when they were beginning to acknowledge that co-dependency is not only a one person problem or a family problem but a societal problem.

Back in 1988 on page 172 Bradshaw states that *"60 million are seriously affected by alcoholism; 60 million are sex abuse victims; 60% are women and 50% are men have an eating disorder; one out of eight is a battered woman; 51% of marriages end in divorce and there is massive child abuse. We are an addicted society. We are severely co-dependent."*

I read that statement and went, "Well that makes sense to me, my mother, my aunt, uncles, and most likely my grandmother, as we are all a part of dysfunctional families and they are more common than fleas on a hairless dog."

I have to make sense of my whole self. I am an avid learner of how to get better, how to grow out of this physical body. (Actualization due to the chapter that I live inside so nothing can hurt me, yet it still does more than ever because of the amount of traumatic events that have occurred since the last triggering.

There are many adjectives/conditions that describe "these children" and may not apply to all persons and they are as follows: abandonment issues, delusion and denial, undifferentiated ego mass, loneliness and isolation, thought disorders. Control madness, hyper vigilant and high levels of anxiety, internalized shame, and lack of boundaries, disabled will, reactive and re-enacting, and numbed out. Offender with or without offender status, fixated personality, dissociated responses, yearning for parental warmth and approval, secrets, faulty communication style, under-involved, neglect of developmental dependency needs, compulsive/addictive, trance- carrying on the family spell, intimacy problems, over-involved, narcissistically deprived, abuse victim, lack of coping skills. False self-confused identity, avoid depression through activity, measured, judgement, and perfectionistic, inhibited trust, loss of your own reality, inveterate dreamer, emotional constraint, and spiritual bankruptcy.

I encourage you to read up on these words because this is your beginning to more personal growth. I find that when it comes to behavioral pattern/thought changing it is often best to read one chapter at a time because reality needs to be addressed in order to move forward.

In the end it does provide solace as you are not alone. In 1988 there was 60 million and the population has increased by a minimum of one; say 30 million more it now brings that to 90 million. We are soon coming up to another minimum 30 million if the growth hasn't already started. Now we are looking at a minimum 120 million people that are "broken". I don't enjoy the word dysfunctional due to the negative perceptional value attached to wording mostly due to the over use in the 80's maybe, but I still have to use the term until "broken" catches on....

Oppositional Defiance Disorder

"Now don't go sticking your finger in the frosting on my freshly baked cake," Mom decreed as she went on to clean something else in anticipation of the surprise party.

The child goes off and plays for a moment or so with his three year old age appropriate toys. He becomes bored and remembers the cake. Like a sly fox, he tiptoes into the kitchen and spies the cake. He looks both ways then takes a big swipe of frosting with his dirty hands, smears it on his face and somehow finds a small tasting entering his mouth, "Mmmmmmmmmmmmmmmm."

Not hearing child-like movement she goes to the kitchen and he says with sad beagle like eyes, "Hee, hee, opps."

The mother can't be angry because hi admission is just too darn cute to scold, therefore she laughs.

The child grows up in the knowledge that he or she can do bad things, get attention for it, and not get into trouble. Hee, hee, opps becomes the reality into everyday life and work settings.

Unless one is aware of this behavior that stemmed from childhood, it does affect lives and environments. It's like a subconscious habit; you are told to do something yet you just can't help yourself from behaving like the three year old child inside and you do the opposite and low and behold you're saying internally, "Hee, hee, opps." Without the admission of this occurrence the emotions of others in the environment become inflamed.

Don't try and convince yourself that nobody knows that it was your three year old self involved and you go merrily on your way. We are adults are we not? Adults "man up" and don't act like the three year old deep inside wanting attention because all he started receiving on a continuous basis was negative attention wanting needs.

Upon acknowledgement of the existence of your child-like behavior it is now time to set things in order by consciously paying attention to our actions. Pretty soon you may just get the positive emotional attention that you've required since you were six month old when you found you were completely dependent on your parents and freaked out whenever you felt "abandoned".

At the Bipolar Checkout

When reading material that helps understand our behaviors, emotions, and thought patterns it can be discerning and falling into a greater depression could occur.

You cannot allow your selves to go there. Trying to be "balanced" about the information is key. Even though it's not the happy, happy, joy, joy moment seeing your selves with the "normality" of society. This is where you can decide whether or not this typical behavior has been helpful or if it needs to be improved upon by "lessening of the emotional problem."

A typical emotional problem that occurs in every broken family is parental abandonment. This comes in the form of consumption of alcohol, and illegal substances of the parent or parents. It can also be emotional abuse, and physical abuse as well where when those situations happen the child feels abandoned.

How does one get over the feeling of abandonment and the idealization of parents that weren't around as often as the vulnerable child required? Your inner child still even as an adult may want the parent or parents as the sense of family security is shattered due to functioning of the family. In order to remove the emotion one needs to acknowledge that it is one of your behaviors, then "dissect" it and like pulling out a sliver; be careful it will hurt.

One may never overcome the abandonment feeling but nothing is instantaneous besides you've just become aware.

Buttons, Everybody Has Them

It has come to my attention that I am blogging about issues that are sensitive but the thing is I wouldn't talk about them if they weren't important and essential in regards to Bipolar Disorder.

When I blog about something, I can be inspired by people I enter-act with and sometimes I blog about experiences I've had in the past and how "getting through it" helped me. Sometimes it may seem like I'm posting something incredibly off but the truth is that I am Bipolar and when I blog or post or do something it is of therapeutic value I share it.

I am trying to blog about something related to Bipolar Disorder every day and sometimes it's hard and sometimes I have to use my emotions and what I'm going through in order for my intent to help the rest of the world who may be in the baby stages of acknowledgement into a flown blown eyes wide open triggering feelings that you thought were hidden from you view.

I would think that it takes a lot of courage to be able to share experiences in a helpful manner. I didn't just arrive at this counseling or helping teach the world what it's like for persons with Bipolar Disorder so that those who don't have it and read this blog will begin to gain some insight on how to help and what it is like.

With so many similarities that we share, know that the blogs aren't about you even if they are hitting that button of yours. If you're mad or hate my blog posting don't be disrespectful and ruin everybody else who reads this site by creating problems with all of the social media outlets I use. They like this website, they read every day what I've written and I cherish that because I know I'm helping someone or people out there in this vast planet.

How to Deal with Your Self

I read this amazing book that helped put my chemically imbalanced self during that time period into a newly moulded set of eyes. The book is called Embracing Our Selves, A Voice Dialogue Manual.

This book talks about the different people we are as we enteract with different people. I say enteract as one word because that is what we are doing; we are entering into an act of a self that is part of our whole "personal makeup" based upon personal repeated exposure, physically and emotionally traumatic events that have occurred during your life.

Say you are 40, it is probable that you are a parent, a brother/sister, aunt/uncle, niece/nephew, child, teacher, co-worker, employee, manager, driver, a grandparent, and the list goes on as you now look at how that self enteracts within that "time frame". This is the typical characteristics of that self dealing with repeated situations and learned experiences.

If you see some behaviors as you replay each "scene" in your head that you are now saying, "What??? Okay, this is a behavioral goal. This is a great step, and one of many as you will grow leaps and bounds acknowledging, saying hello to each self, and allowing that self to "speak".

It may seem "loco" but it does work. It works better so you don't appear so "craaazzeee" with somebody that you trust. As each self "appears" be that self and sit where that self would sit because you can't sit in the same place for each self. This is where your subconscious physical body acknowledges the presence of a self. I worked on this by myself as I was watching a movie in my brain and it turns into a frequent behavioral check method because as persons with Bipolar Disorder we do have to "monitor" our selves because well, "we" as Bipolars tend to get into trouble, at least that's what we think for whatever we've done that at that moment in our mind it just seemed okay to do that. It could be "correct" or it could be "incorrect" it really is dependent on which "self" you are being because remember we can be the "bad cop" self; over admonishing our selves for something that in reality is inconsequential and the enteracting party didn't even notice.

There may come a moment when you may start thinking that you have multiple personalities and you better check yourself into the institution but the reality is that every person on this planet has multiple selves just like you but are now aware and in the land of acknowledgement.

When your self becomes scared or starts crying, let it. It is necessary to let this self express them self in this manner. Talk it out with your trust partner but only that self at that moment and as soon as another self appears change places and let that self express because you are going to find the one that protects you, the one that defends you, the victim, and once you "go there" you'll never want to go back to the land of blissfulness again.

You have enhanced your life. Or just starting to enhance your life. One thing I would like to point out that everybody knows and forgets at the same time, is that at the two week mark of changing your selves into a better person you will want to "fall back" on the old because these new ones are "too hard, it's not helping" and if those are some words you are saying, I'll return to you with,

"You're not trying hard enough. If I can change my life around you can too. It all starts with the selves."

The Simplest of Things in Life

Have you ever had one of those days where you just relaxed and did nothing all day? Most people can afford to enjoy doing nothing, persons with any type of Bipolar Disorder this can be a constant state when depressed. Day after day after day we drown in the simplest of tasks from lack of "will"; lack of drive. You see it, you acknowledge it then you slump in hopelessness and still don't accomplish the simplest of tasks like loading a dishwasher.

Yes, the simplest of tasks, those mundane tasks that you have no problem accomplishing because you are in a "high drive" state without the use of medication. But yet even on medication there can be the down periods of feeling overwhelmed because you see the windows need to be cleaned, dusting, vacuuming, sweep, and mop the floor. Don't even get started on talking about doing laundry because that's almost a major feat in itself where you get into the watching machine and forget about it until the next day or an improvement is transferring it over to the dryer and the start button pushed. A really good day consists of transfer into a laundry basket and a minimum of two loads accomplished.

I know that normal people think that this is just laziness but I have found we are like waves; up, down, gently, swiftly, a tidal wave and one that crashes upon the shoreline.

I am an advocate of persons with a type of Bipolar Disorder to have access and if there is obtain the help of a Residential Care Aid that is specifically to help people like me because, like everyone else I have a hard time doing the simplest of tasks. I am extremely lucky to have a supportive and loving husband who doesn't mind if I don't do the dishes for three days even though it should only take fifteen minutes at the most to accomplish the task. I could go on about the support he does provide but like most people he has to work so there's a vast amount of time when we're by ourselves wanting to do something but having an anxiety attack about doing it our self.

There in itself can lead to a depressive state. The want to do something like landscaping, chopping wood, fishing, attending to serious matters but need some help. Alas there is none is to be found and the want to ask for help from friends and family isn't an option to due to the fear of being told no or that they are busy because well, that's the thing about life is that everybody has one and their time is spent elsewhere. One cannot expect family and friends to drop everything for you, even though you need the support. This is where the Residential Care Aid comes in. If you need support they are there. That's their job; to help you get the things done that need to be attended to but as a team.

Extended Health Insurance Corporations and Clients

It has come to my attention that if one was on welfare or Income Assistance that all of your health needs are looked after and there is little to no money out of pocket in British Columbia. It is true that persons of very low income can get free eye exams that cost $80 and go to the chiropractor for $11.

I'm not sure why Medical Insurance companies stopped at (according to research so far) Dentists for providing instant access of the client's Extended Health Benefits where the insurance portion is automatically deducted and the client pays the remaining on the day of service.

One train of thought that the Extended Health Benefit Provider is that if one can afford to pay for the extended health that they can afford to pay $80 for the eye exam and $50 to see the chiropractor.

You see the system is set up that the client pays up front and then submits a claim form and sends it into the insurance company for the refundable portion. When you buy glasses on Income Assistance you don't pay a dime for them but if you have Extended Health Benefits you pay the full amount and submit the form to be reimbursed.

Sometimes companies provide the extended health by deducting the monthly cost off the employee's pay cheque therefore making it appear as though one can afford to fully pay for much needed health related services.

Recently I found out that Optometry (eye doctor) exams the client has to pay up front the complete cost. I talked to the ladies behind the desk and chatted about how one could have it set up that insurance companies worked with their health service. I told them I'd get back to them and so I called my extended health care provider and ask why or if it was possible and the customer service person said we don't have anything set up right now to do that. Please go to our website and suggest it. So I did.

The thing that confuses me the most is according my perception of the phone call is that no one has ever questioned "The System" in regards to seeing the eye doctor every three years like one is "supposed to" being able to afford contacts/glasses. I don't know about you but with the cost of gas, groceries, rent, electric, heat, loan/credit card payments I don't see how middle income persons can afford to pay for these services upfront and be able to afford to live while waiting for the refundable portion.

If everyone made this suggestion to the Extended HealthCare Insurance Providers then change can being and have Health Service be connected to these corporations who make millions of dollars a year taking client payments, never lacking money nor trying to figure when they can afford to see the Eye Doctor or Chiropractor because they can afford to wait for their refund.

I have financial anxieties which makes it feel like I can never afford to buy the glasses I need to wear or to have the eye exam that I've been needing to have for the last five years and having Bipolar Disorder, well I haven't been in.

While I'm thinking about it; the prescription system should be changed as well because well, I'm paying upfront for all that and my medication is important, (I have to take it) and again my financial anxieties are triggered.)

Patterns, Choices, Abilities; the Societal Viewpoint

Where, O, where do you begin with people/society and their constant use of foul language/language unbecoming of from even the filthiest of mouths? Seriously, it is getting ridiculous out there and there are far better words to be used when expressing angry emotions that is like the song "Hokey, Pokey" and yes, the world may think it is ridiculous to say such words, "flippr doonjaa" instead of the good old fashioned "f u c k". Another expression is "frosted flakes and cheerios" instead of "son of a b i t c h". While "bajigglee wiggle" is frowned upon yet it is far better to hear than "f u c k i n g w h o r e" even if it is an object not a person.

It is an everyday common occurrence and acceptable levels of toleration grow as society seems to lack the ability to use a thesaurus or a dictionary for that matter. Does anyone remember the expression, "If you don't have anything nice to say don't say anything at all?" I'd like to rephrase it; "If all you can do is spew out foul language then be quiet." The world doesn't need you to add to the "garbage" out there.

I do not believe that there is one perfect person out there. I do believe however, that we have the ability to choose and make choices. We have the ability to be remorseful. We have unlimited abilities; it is THE CHOICE THAT IS MADE that is the outcome; what the world sees.

Does the world see you screaming, yelling, carrying on over the minutest of things or does the world see you advocating on wrong doings; bring forth attention that is much needed in this society that creeps into the dirtiest of business practices and yet, the world says this is "okay" while this person does not think that it is okay and will say so.

When we carry on like hyenas it is often only heard as screaming "raaaaaarrrrraaaaaaaaaarrrrrrrrrrrrrrraaaaaaaaaa" and overwhelming excessive profanity which by political correctness needs to be forgiven by the one that has been desecrated; God.

Does anybody realize that He is always watching? He sees you when you are sleeping. He sees you when you are awake and He knows when you've been bad or good so you better watch out because God as we all know prefers to be praised and profanity is not praising Him at all. Reading the Bible is going to church doesn't count for redemption. It is based upon correcting the behavior and acting just like Jesus did when they flogged him, and nailed him to the cross; he took it and he let the people do their "sinful" act so that he could save us all.

Now if I was in his shoes well, and I saw this excessive use I would be infuriated as one could be reciting Proverbs instead. I am not Jesus but I do try to be good in this unjustly world I live in. There are many wolves waiting out there and they come in all shapes and forms. It is our choice to emanate a behavior and it is our choice to find a different means of expression or a completely different behavior that is more suitable for "societal viewing".

If behavioral changes was meant to be easy then we'd all be able to wear our "Happy Helmets" and everybody would get along.

I've had ten years of trying to consistently wear my "Happy Helmet" although unappreciated by others.

Even though I've read lots of self-help books, have taken a counseling course I do fall very short of perfection but as a person who is willing to look at events and correct behaviors, and move forward I'm doing "pretty good". I'm not doing fantastic but that would mean an escalation in my want of "mind evolution of thought patterns" and helping others go beyond this very topic of excessive use of   profane   words.

Financial Anxieties and Where They Can Take You

One of the things about being a Counselor according to the Skilled Helper is that as a Counselor one must be "willing to go there". If a person doesn't have an experience that another has described how is it that once can begin to understand the depths that an anxiety will drive a person under-medicated to that has a type of Bipolar Disorder?

From the depths of being raised in a "well-off" family. Although it didn't seem like it or was given the appearance that the family had a sufficient amount of money to fulfill each want without getting a loan or some material object to going to the food bank every week to obtain one weeks' worth of food. One time I even walked from the old Expo '86 building all the way up Kingsway to 41st and Wales in East Vancouver back in 1993 when I was 17 years old just to go to the central food bank locations as the other was closed. I lived in some pretty hard times but fun times. I don't recall fighting with my boyfriend. When I had a job I was good with my money and we didn't seem to lack. Back then I took the transit systems that are available.

When I moved back to my home town I got a minimum wage job and started working. Again here I am 18 years old living on my own with and without a boyfriend. By the time I was 19 years old I was married, and by the age of 20 had my only child. During the course of ten years I had several minimum wage paying jobs and a couple of better paying jobs. We made ends meet and most of the time the ends didn't meet and something was sold like my full mount cougar, the full mount coyote, one full mount black bear that was made "Limpy", a grizzly bear rug, several rifles, racked up the credit cards, lost a car due to the inability to make payments, got in "too deep" with credit and I had to declare bankruptcy.

Feeling unhappy and the repeated exposure situations that kept occurring I left and for six months lived on less than $900 per month. I had to have room-mates and well we'll say that they weren't the best choices I have made but back then I was un-medicated due to financial anxieties about affording them. We live where we can afford to live at least that's what occurred when I moved into a town house location where more often than not there persons living there were low income. Now there is nothing wrong with being low income. I've been there, I've done it. You learn to how to be effective with your money, you also begin to feel that you never can afford to buy anything and never be able to afford to get ahead, never be anything because it takes money to make money.

Now I have tried to be self-employed and if I had money or working capital I would be successful and I wouldn't still be suffering from Financial Anxieties but I am getting back the loads of books that I have written since about 1996. I just found another one today because my publisher was talking about publishing a cookbook and I said, "I have one of those". It is funny how life works; I have been trying to obtain a self-employment loan to become self-published with full color illustrations, buying books, going on an Author Tour would cost $50 000 to finding out I could self-publish for free almost eight years later.

During those eight years I kept trying to find a way to obtain funds to fulfil this want of being published, being the success that I know is mine to be had, the goals that have been listed on a poster board so that when I forget what I'm doing I can look at it and remind myself to "Keep Moving Forward". For every mistake there is lesson to be learned. Back in 2010 I acknowledged some very unbecoming feeling and an age condition that was causing fights in a relationship so I left. A very grievous mistake was made by the other party leaving a feeling obligation. I was desperate. I needed money to pay off every single debt that was outstanding; to rectify and be able to leave because every wrong would have been righted. Of course during this time period I sold my car, a 4 wheeler was sold too quickly due to impulsiveness son some persons' part, I've tried to get on Dragon's Den two times, emailed several daytime talk shows trying to get help for the book that is now called Junior Hunters at Large and I will not forget that I emailed them at least 3 times. Ones that I remember are as follows: Ellen, Oprah, Montel Williams, Dr. Keith O'Blow, Tyra Banks, and even Howie Mandel. I never received a response from any of them. I'm wondering if they'd have me now that I have 6 books published and still moving through the depression, the good times, the forced happiness, financial anxieties, and many other factors that are part of my living, breathing, and "Keep Moving Forward" attitude. I have been involved in a 419 scam where a wolf rug, a cougar rug was sold for "paying" to obtain funds. Loan payments were ceased to be made and every person involved had their credit go down the tube once more because I had this need to have money so I could start this life that somehow doesn't show who I am inside.

Almost four year later, things are picking up but then it seems to fall to pieces upon revelations that have occurred without full disclosure on both sides. I finally have the ability to repair all the credit damage done so that a mortgage approval would be made in about 14 months if enough money was saved but the payment is at an excessive percentage that making the loan payment a "holy doodle" scare me to death; I have Financial Anxieties and very unsure about the stability of my life.

The word "stuck" is often used by those who want out of a relationship or are very unhappy with the conditions that they are "enduring" but then we are encountered with not having enough money to "get unstuck" without asking for help from others. I've been there; I've gone back to the paternal home, stayed at others places for a few days, and lived in a travel trailer once for three months trying to pay off all debts outstanding from leaving the low income town house area. I've asked parental help to leave, asked relatives and have received help, asked friends, I even tried to explain how relationships are nowadays to grandparents and have had roommates oh and I have asked my ex-husband.

In marriages that suffer from financial discourse it is often best to see the whole picture and how it can be solved, at least that is my perception of trying to solve financial discourse. If person A says "Get a job" person B says "Okay I will, but will there be a vehicle available to me instead of taking the bus? Do we have enough money for me to take the bus until a pay period occurs? When do you start applying for a job? Is that on the Friday that a cheque arrives or should I wait until Monday? Are you on afternoons for two weeks when there is money or are you on dayshift now? Which day of the week do you have off? Can I use the vehicle to go to the doctors' instead and have pills that help lessen depression? Do you have anything planned on your day off that requires the vehicle that is winter drive-able?"

With all the questions is it any wonder that Financial Anxieties exist? Even though these questions are rather specific some can be thought of as generic; the typical Bipolar Disordered person who has Financial Anxieties which affects and effects every aspect of their life. Many seem to think that being home all day is fun except it isn't fun when you feel "stuck".

Please Come Fill the Gap

There has been a steady stream on Canada's channels about how an American cellphone company provider wants to come to Canada. Although 81% said no, I say yes.

Why? First off there would no longer be inadequate cellphone coverage across Canada as I have stated in blogs about how we live in a social media world and the lack of it can create an Internet Withdrawal Syndrome.

Internet Withdrawal Syndrome is when somebody is used to having the convenience of using a cellphone or internet and experience poor quality cellphone/internet service or no cellphone/internet service at all. Some may experience this type of syndrome due to loss of usage of either breakage/repair/lost. This syndrome can be felt within moments of loss or inability to use a cellphone or internet. It does not cease until the ability to use the services is available once more. Each day or time that a person tries to use this type of "service" and experiences negative repeated exposure, the anger level of emotion increases.

Acknowledging the numbers for person with a type of Bipolar Disorder on this planet ranges from 2 000 000 to 80 000 000 we can afford to "trigger" these people as they have challenges in functioning in everyday life. Most persons with a type of Bipolar Disorder are usually Social Media orientated as a form of socializing as most don't interact within the "physical location" area of where they are residing. You will find them at home depressive/anticipation period.

So I ask that the United States cellphone corporation(s) push forward with this added information about Bipolar Disorder so that the "triggering" will be reduced. I know that you will share the towers with the Canadian corporations as they seem to lack the funds to provide complete coverage. This way every corporations wins.

The second most important, in my opinion, is that hopefully the monthly/prepaid plan costs will be reduced drastically. There will be more GB for the price which will be lower than the current average price rate. I've seen Verizon, Cellular.com showing low rate availability which will make it affordable for everyone who can't afford the luxurious top of the line cellphone.

Welcome to Canada on behalf of all persons who have a type of Bipolar Disorder. We look forward to the relief of constant "triggering" of I.W.S. (Internet Withdrawal Syndrome).

I am a happy Telus Mobility Smart Hub customer but I'd like more "airwave" coverage.

The Option to Grow, Care for Ones' Self, and to Self-Nurture

When we get down to the basics of any relationships we tend to find ourselves in a triangle and what is termed by Stephen Karpman as the Drama Triangle which consists of a Persecutor, Rescuer, and a Victim.

I would like to relate to this relate as the base to recognize Repeated Exposure. If you think back to every relationship you have been in (thinking more along the lines of intimate relationships) which role you have been; have you been the Persecutor (they like to emotionally drain you with verbally abusive words and they like to be in control of everything) or have you been the Rescuer (you know the one who is always helping the "poor me's" consistently) or are you the Victim?

When you take the perception and look at the word victim and how it applies to you, what is it or what was it that created the "Victim" Self? How many times have you been in that type of situation? There's your repeated exposure thus explaining the emotional rise when "triggered" by ordinary events.

What if your role is what others perceive you to be the Victim while the whole time you're angry with yourself for taking this role, angry about the helpless feelings, and you know your True Self.

I've been told that most relationships are like this; a "Hold You Down" due to fear and anxieties of the partner, the "I Am Doing as I Learned Watching", or the "I Am Going to

Save You". This is normal. What you can do to break this triangle is to start to be proactive and empower yourself to being in better mental health.

I can offer two sides to this coin due to being the one being counseled and from a counselors' perspective with repeated exposure to proactive trying and they are as follows:

21 Day Rule: You have 21 days to be constant/diligent of writing down feelings that surface when you think about your wants; going to the grocery store, wanting to do more marketing but are afraid of being rejected or looking unprofessional due to thought patterns that it is far more professional to have someone calling on behalf than to be making the calls/emails/requests/messages etc.

(Okay so that's my issue and it's a tough one that I will be going through. It's hard for me because of the hunting and fishing industry and my book Junior Hunters at Large. I've experienced negative repeated exposure to trying to get help with promotion as this is an excellent book promoting kids to go hunting and fishing. I don't feel comfortable posting a link to my book on their hunting and fishing pages.)

So if you look at being proactive in overcoming this hurdle is that positive emotional support from the support network to show the "I Believe in You" is very helpful and encouraging "It's Time to Work" moments.

When you are feeling up or down in feeling you need to record this so that you can begin to see a pattern. When you start feeling down; ask yourself what happened? Were you the Victim again? If you were then this is the first step to becoming aware and that's the first movement to change.

Repeated Exposure Triggering

One of things about being a counselor is that we are taught to divert attention to a different aspect when the client is trying to discuss feeling about what is happening for them. Once could say that on average this works as long as there is not an extended period of repeated exposure. If a person has had less than 3 weeks (21 days) of a trigger this diversion is achievable and also dependent upon the willingness of the client to move forward.

When a client has had more than 21 days but less than 365 it will take more to remove the trigger versus trying to divert their attention. It takes even more effort from the counselor and the client to resolve the triggers that creates the emotional level. The counselor should not try to redirect onto what the "True Self" is up to when work is in progress.

More often than not I've experienced this type of counseling before and it's not that effective for extended long term repeated exposure. As a person who has a trigger that is out of control due to 1 825 days passing and no resolution to be told that we need to talk about something else is like trying to sweep dirt under the rug; at the end of the day it is still there unresolved. You can talk until you are blue in the face to someone about all the things that are "okay" with the situation or "it's not uncommon" as the "spoon full of sugar that helps the medicine go down" remedy but the reality for that person is you sound like Charlie Browns' teacher and you have lost your client.

It can be quite difficult to deal with someone who has been triggered within a day of a counseling session. I know that I am not an easy client because I keep being cut off from what needs to be talked about. The thing about calendars and when you put marks on them for when you are triggered you get to see a pattern. In my case I'm seeing someone else's pattern of behavior. Others may not see it this way but they are not looking at it from the correct perspective; the mark means a trigger occurred and what it was. I see a two week pattern of nothingness and then my trigger starts up again. The thing we are told is that we are choosers of our world; so if we choose to sit on a couch and whine and snivel about our lives we are choosing that, if we say we can't do something we are then "disabling" ourselves and are no longer able to take function with that skill. We choose our lives, we can choose to be happy, we can choose to be sad, we can choose to be angry, and we can also choose to be a pity pot. See that is how it works, when you choose it, therefore creates a reaction from the persons whom you are trying to obtain attention from.

While others may see certain issues as laughable, out of control, baffled, or confusing, they are the ones who forget that they haven't experienced the repeated exposure. They are new; like fresh born babies saying this and that like cooing to an infant who isn't an infant and it's pretty angry when people are "cooing" at it. You can't "sing nursery rhymes", you have to talk about the trigger then when it is resolved or exhausted then you can move forward because at the end of the day the emotional range should be less and therefore able to move forward to having a better day.

The other step is complete trigger removal to remove yourself completely from whatever it is that is triggering your emotions because at the end of the day there are usually two emotions left; "I'm tired of this and I need to change it" and or "I'm happy and I have no triggers" but then again that is in a land where fluffy animals, balloons, rainbows, and sunshine play all day or is there a real world where a person can be happy without being triggered?

I Try Not to See You, You See Me

"It's hard to explain to someone who has no clue. It's a daily struggle being in pain or feeling sick on the inside while you look fine on the outside.

Please share this message on your Facebook wall if you, or someone you know has an invisible illness: Crohn's, PTSD, Anxiety, Depression, Fibromyalgia, Bipolar, Lupus, MS, ME, Arthritis, Cancer, Heart Disease, Epilepsy, Muscular Dystrophy, Autism etc.

Never judge what you don't understand." – Anonymous

One of the greatest achievements in my opinion for persons with a type of Bipolar Disorder is the ability to survive enter-actions. I say enter-actions because of the simple fact that as I walk through a door, I have now entered and here comes the actions of every single person in the store making whiplash movement to the jingling bell advising of someone coming into the store.

It can be one of life's greatest anxieties for some that do not enjoy being stared at due to an obscene amount of unwanted staring

Maybe today wasn't the best of days for me, but the thing is that every person who has this type of anxiety, this is what it's like. I also have to keep reminding myself that I live in a small town and this is the way they have been since the Goldrush period back in the 1860's. So I exaggerate a little, it's to make the point that every single place of business where I walk through the door and the exact same thing occur; The Whiplash Movement, and how annoying it is that this is a subconscious behavior that simply seems to be "acceptable" by the rest of society who does not have this type of anxiety or a type of Bipolar Disorder for that matter.

It is quite common to see me walk through a door looking like a stone wall giving the impression that I may be a snob but that is just because of your favorite activity; staring. I guess we could walk through the door and stare at you like, "OH MY GOODNESS WHAT IS THAT!!!" That's just one thought that is running through our minds as we try to navigate quickly to where we want to be seated or making a purchase decision. **********************AND IT FEELS LIKE YOU ARE ALL STARING AT ME STILL***************** I am like everybody else who wants to be left alone from the peering, leering eyes. I am not staring at you, I am trying to do some shopping.

We could be Mystery Shoppers, you never know, or maybe Muncipal By-Law Enforcement as you have a dog in your place of business that is not a Seeing Eye Dog that just went outside and took a poop (yup only in a small town) and was let in immediately. I don't mean to be rude but if you are going to have your maybe you could buy them "wipeys" and wipe their bums for them because I nearly puked. I hope they wash the carpet the dog lays on every day because you know, they could… and really I am sure we all have an imagination about what dogs do when they drag their bum across the floor or lawn…

Does anyone else have a problem with this? Or is this just another "Bipolar Disorder" thing?

Remembering that everybody is somebody, that's right, somebody. We are CUSTOMERS, we have money to spend, and we are in your store for a reason. I do not know why you seem to forget that, seriously you are paid to provide proper business ethical conduct, you are to be informative, you are to be acknowledging the fact that products and services are expensive and therefore saving customers money is important, AND YOU DO NOT SELL OUTDATED PRODUCTS. If you don't have good business ethics don't expect me to shop there and I will say something about it.

The sad part is that this type of activity occurs all over the world and the sick thing is, at least in my opinion, that society accepts this as normal. It is because of my condition that I am and we are more prone to say something like I did today when I was cut-off by people that couldn't just wait three second for us to pass so they could enter their store. I let them go first and said, "That's all right I'm not in that big of a hurry." Or when we were at the furniture store and the TV Display area they had on the sales floor was dusty with no price tags. The only model available to purchase at that time unless one wants to wait two weeks. (What's with that anyways? Why is that they cannot keep one or two models in the back? Does your staff know how to order products when they have sold one? It does not appear to be so.) I said, "I'm not that desperate." We went to another store and I will not go back again because that was just nasty, I was gagging in the parking lot because somebody brings their pet in to work and well the whole dog poo smell. The topper to this place was yet again, they did not have the TV we wanted in stock. I couldn't handle the smell, I went outside had a smoke, drank my specialty coffee and waited then I got tired and I walked through the door and WHIPLASH MOVEMENT to learn that my husband that does love me very much is settling for the display model and I say, "Is it gold plated, are you getting extra warranty with that? Is that what is taking so long? I have to keep reminding myself that this is 100 Mile."

It is not that we look for problems but if you have, like me, a problem with people who do not know how to provide quality customer service, conduct unethical business practice/conduct we will not like you. Due to our condition we stand up and say something. If you encounter me, be grateful I take medications so I am less than I would be if I didn't. If you encounter a person who has a type of Bipolar Disorder and isn't taking medication they' be yelling and screaming. It's not a normal habit for me to yell and scream, if I have, you've really triggered me and I am expressing myself clearly. But then again, I'm pretty sure that all persons with a type of Bipolar Disorder acknowledged or unacknowledged act like this.

I Advocate for Bipolar Disorder Awareness please remember   that.

True Stories; the Life Blood of Inspiration for Creators

I am an inspirational true story DVD collector. They are usually found alphabetically in their category which of course is obviously titled "True Stories" that I like to watch when "all hope seems lost" or when I've had a recent dousing of the "normality" that persons that are creative experience. You know that feeling; embarking upon the precipice, feeling good, on the rise and then wham it happens. Somewhere out there is a voice, the discorded one, the pessimistic joy of tear down.

One of the things I've learned about these types of situations is that when there is an occurrence it is usually because there is jealousy, envy, and some levels of anger towards the one that is creating. If a creator did not create what would they do?

Did you know that 80% of persons who have a type of mental illness enjoy consuming alcoholic beverages? Did you know that there are more than 80 000 000 people in the world that admit to having a type of Bipolar Disorder? Personally, I don't find the statistic scary. What I do find scary is the amount of people in the world who have this condition or type of mental illness that don't acknowledge that they have a chemical imbalance because that is all it is. You take an emotion, repeated exposure to situations, the chemical imbalance and what you get is an outburst, a show "I" ness, as they prance like the tiny devils that they are.

Now in the movies that I own and watch it clearly shows that there are people who like to "hold down", "trash", and any other word that can describe the "brick wall" feeling that helps create depression. In those movies the creators pick themselves up and they keep going.

I watch movies about segregation and how white people treated other. It amazes me that a color should affect the value of an individual and yet it sill occurs in this world. Actually it takes place every day and sometimes it's not even a skin color discrimination. It can be a labeling a societal, perceptional views, and opinions. Life offers a variety of reasons to pass judgement but if we are to pass judgement in life how is it that we can function in our daily lives or are we function on passing judgements?

If the creator of the intermittent wiper gave up when all hope seemed lost we would never know how corporations take ideas away from creators. Or how about the amount of persecution during the racist times, if they did not break down the barrier and keep moving forward where would we be at on an intellectually aware level that some things that happen in life aren't right but those people who kept "plugging away" despite all the negativity that surrounded them didn't go and do a smear campaign as their victory march. They worked harder and I'm betting that even though they were breaking down "walls" that they often felt like all hope was lost and just maybe they had inspirational stories that kept reminding them to keep moving forward.

I've read the book Touched with Fire; The Manic Depressive Illness and the Artistic Temperament by Dr. Kay Redfield Jamieson where she has lists of and lists of poets, musicians, scriptwriters, political persons that like to drink, and do other substances and they are highly regarded as the author of the book lists "symptoms" and behaviors.

Needless to say, take hear creators, know that you are not alone, and if you ever feel like all hope is lost watch an inspirational true story and then, keep moving forward.

Recommended Titles:

The Blind Side, Faith Like Potatoes, Julie & Julia, Against the Ropes, Seabiscuit, Flash of Genius, Pride, Defiance, The Gridiron Gang, Secretariat, Freedom Writers, Glory Road, We Are Marshall, Swimming Upstream, Hidalgo

Attention #Psychiatrist, #Psychologists, #All Medical Personnel

I do apologize for the # tags but it's the only way you are going to know the correct and proper procedures for dealing, caring for persons with a type of Mental Illness or even going through Withdrawal Symptoms requiring help.

"The Mental Illness Admission Act and Procedure
Effective Feb/10/2014"

Author: Terri Kovalcik

1. If client claims needing into crisis stabilization record all information as per standard regulatory procedure.
2. Ask if this is a "REPEATED EXPOSURE SITUATION"
   Definition of Repeated Exposure: where an occurrence of any sort has continued to happen with negative result for more than two weeks. If the answer is no, ask how long. Ask what the repeated exposure issue is.
3. Place phone call to crisis stabilization center and advise of their new ward. SHIFT CHANGE IS CANCELLED. THE CLIENT IS MORE IMPORTANT THAN GABBING ABOUT PERSONAL THINGS)
4. If there is a waiting period do not allow that person to be around other persons. Your client has a type of Mental Illness that does not allow proper function in social environments waiting 10 hours plus just to get into the best care facility in the South Cariboo. Give these

clients an isolating room until they are received by the proper facility.

5. When calling the facility the code word I'd like to recommend is CODE TLC (which means tender loving care) write that on the bracelets so everybody knows that this person requires TLC regardless of grumpy levels first thing in the morning.

6. Whenever possible refer to the Royal Inland Hospital "Section S" they have a wonderful staff, excellent and caring patients who bond together supporting each other. They are located in Kamloops, British Columbia. Do not send them to the emergency ward at your local hospital that is not equipped to deal with CODE TLC's. (I, Terri Kovalcik, fully support and endorse without proper consent.)

I would like to recommend that a Massage Therapist be on hand so that all the muscles can be relaxed from soreness that is an effect of the conditions from whatever your TLC has. I've seen soothing warm rocks rubbed in a soothing fashion on a client's back; it's all about calming the client down, and the first step to showing part of the emotional love without prejudice they could receive. Also laptops be available for social media/Facebook purposes because it's hard enough getting better without a social network that loves and worries about you as well. When in the ward they can learn how to "tap" their creativity. There are Facebook mental health groups that many would benefit from.

I would also like to ask that Quetapine and Lithium be banned from being prescribed to persons with Bipolar Disorder. These people are creative and if they were able to focus on doing something that makes them smile versus being lethargic and please excuse the bluntness, but a complete waste of talent.

I would like to recommend a "REAL" Counselor for persons with Bipolar Disorder because according to The Skilled Helper textbook from ICS Learn is one who has BIPOLAR DISORDER (which is me. Please feel free to pay me per visitation, I'd be happy to stay at the unit while I'm able to help.)

Imagine if Charles Dickens, Winston Churchill, Mozart, William Shakespeare, Robert Frost, Stephen King were all on Lithium (the max dosage because that the favorite starting point *perceptually* you wouldn't any books to read. I'm going to bet you a dollar for a donut that Gene Rodenberry, one of my all-time inspirers of the creators of the Science Fiction Genre. What if he was given medication where a side effect is that you almost drool all day every day? Would he still be considered one of the Literary Greats? Our Literary Greats wouldn't have written a thing, they would have ended up in the "they're useless society" and let's see if we can drill a hole into their brain and see what's wrong. Opps they did already did that. How did   that   work   out   anyways?

The Words That Flowed While Under

While waiting in the emergency room in Kamloops, not really coherent to the rest of the world, I opened one of my notebooks and with pen in hand, customized of course, these words appeared, staying forever as there is a message I am sure.

If I was to draw a map it would be a weaving circle that never ends through all the loops and holes, the overs and unders, climbing the wall; the impenetrable wall that will never come down. It is the fear of acknowledgement it is a place that most don't want to see or acknowledge the existence of what they have become.

The Mobius strip offers us many opportunities to experience things over and over again but in a new way, a different approach because the Mobius strip is always turning, looping and a piece of tape is all that holds it together.

As time passes the glue becomes dry, the tape tatters excessive turning and all that is left is a dirty piece of paper that shows the over usage of the Mobius strip.

If one could be a piece of paper and a pencil was used to write on it, all the mistakes could be erased.

The wave crashes on the shore, white foam leaves its path where it has been and where it went. The foamy reef takes and gathers all from everywhere it exits taking from one area leaving a piece at another. The foam is light, wavy, bubbly, toiling with intricate seaweeds immersing themselves into a vegetable kelp salad.

Tendrils of life the seaweed flows, the weaving, fans in a stadium enjoying each nation the flow the journey it takes upon the ocean water everywhere but not a drop to drink.

The life blood of human; water if waters is the life of human how is it that we can survive without a drop to drink. Do we pray for the water? When the water comes do we pray in hatred for it to stop?

And when desire comes, do you strike a match to light the way or do we make blazing fire for all to see?

Fire, water, air, and life is what we've been given so where along the way did we miss the bus and this is the final stop.

It is the whine-ness you say, we must go, there's more to this life and it will be as making pie.

The easier it looks to make a perfect pie one has to have mode. Over a hundred times just to get one perfect pie.

The Turn-Over Rate

Have you ever watched people? I watch all the time and I see all kinds of things as I cast glances here and there driving, stopping, "consumerizing" myself with needs and wants shopping at various locations and shops. I love travelling, it's a great way to see the world other than just the town you live in. You can experience all kinds of things while out and about.

There will be places that you'll never go back to because it needs some help in some form or another. It could be the food or the customer service or it could the ambience. There are places that you tell everybody about. At least I do because if it's awesome and you see me there then you know it's worthy of your money to be spent there. If I don't shop there then there is a reason.

As a person with a type of Bipolar Disorder I have a list of not unusual anxieties which are when we are working in the customer service industry dealing with grumpy people, people who have children acting out, and most importantly fellow co-workers.

I have to say that some of my favorite lines that I will never forget because I personally thought it was ridiculous in comparison to my emotional roller coaster past but I was happy at work, I told jokes at work, I woke up at 5:30am just to hear the joke of the day on Comedy Club 54 thus providing smiling happy faces at the workplace. Now this person who is nameless said, "I cry every night because my 80 year old boyfriend won't marry me." Yes somebody said that and here I am at that time already tried to "take myself out of existence and here she is 40 complaining about that?" That was the end for me there. Actually that was the end of me working, period. I had been in the employment race 13 years in the customer service industry experiencing similar and new types of negative repeated exposure. Not everybody gets to be as fortunate as I am. There other 80 000 000 people out there who acknowledge their condition also endure this. It is everywhere and it's irritating quite frankly.

I do look at the wanted ads every once in 1a while and I see the same businesses hiring. Potential causes for this turnover rate:

1. The employer has less than desirable business ethics/business practice.
2. The people that work there have been there for an extended period of time and they have the "attitude" to go with it.
3. The co-workers talk about their personal lives at work while serving customers.
4. The use of a cellphone/smartphone lives at work while serving customers.
5. Poor customer service skills.
6. Co-workers talking about customers in a less than desirable fashion in front of other customers.
7. Co-workers talking about other co-workers at work in front of customers.

These are just some of the things that starts my emotional flare and the silly thing is that it bothers others but they don't say anything. Why is that? Do we live in a society where if you treat your customers badly they will continue to shop there because there is nowhere else to shop other than in another town? I am not ashamed to admit that I do shop out of town and I have heard several "consumerizing" complaints because I talk about Bipolar Disorder everywhere I go.

So the next time you are "consumerizing" watch the lines up at the tills, see the peoples' faces, what are they doing? Watch the door to see the look of shock on their faces as they see three tills open with five or more people and more arriving and one express lane with about seven waiting and more coming. Now look at the employees, what are they doing? Look for the person and charge and see what they are doing.

Do you think this is a good turnover rate for productivity? McDonalds, and Tim Hortons have standards for turnover rates, I would like to think that all franchise businesses do too. So are you going to stand there just like everybody else or are you going to say something and change it for the   I

Consequences for the Listening Entrepreneurial Bipolar Disordered

In the "land of" Bipolar Disorder one typically finds the un-medicated, under-medicated, and the "Bull" who does not listen to ideas presented. You can see them in supervisors, managers, employees who have worked at the same job for an extended period of time. These behaviors that we have of not listening takes the form of words like, "No, it works this way. You can't do that because this is how it works. No I can't afford that. I find this extremely hard to imagine." Such words are these given the constant reminder that persons with a type of Bipolar Disorder are stubborn and will not take the advice of others.

If the person with a type of Bipolar Disorder has evolved to thinking about ideas presented and deciding whether or not it is "worthy of their time" to take on such an activity or financial task. Typically speaking, touched with fire persons don't have a large income and everything seems like a financial mountain to overcome so when we "get there" it has cost us much more than what the "blissful" person who encouraged an activity because money slides into their hand far faster than ours and the amount they receive is probably three to four times more than somebody such as myself.

One of the things that needs to be remember is the person with the type of Bipolar Disorder has anxieties, and repeated exposure situations. It may not seem like much to you that they are in front of you but it has taken them a large amount of courage to even want to interact within the geographical location they are residing in.

If you live in your hometown, people do treat you differently and people have to like you if you are deemed "prestigious" or worthy of being nice to. Now if you are an "immigrant" (somebody who does not originate from the town of their new residence) these "home-Towner's" don't have to be nice and they don't have to be nice to the tourists because they are not of "their town" and for some odd reason they are unable to connect customers to money that keeps their stores or businesses open. Through the years the touched with fire individual will emerge and those who deemed the immigrant unworthy is now not enjoy the flourish "ment" and to be beyond their "living society".

The most important point to be made is that persons with a type of Bipolar Disorder are affected emotionally despite any type of medication, so the more negative repeated exposure they receive, the angrier they get. It is often best to let them "present" then just be quiet because when we listen that's when we tend to run into problem after problem trying to "follow through" with your idea.

Oh sure, we can dress up fancy, look like a million dollars when presenting in public but truthfully the share sheds are where I find my clothes because sometimes I buy them. I am "cheap" but with an eye for quality like most of us learn to be. There is a saying that is extremely old but needs to be brought forth; "Never judge a book by its cover." This can be a problematic situation as one can see; dressing professionally but lacking capital to work from. I ended up at the pawn shop where I pawned off my camera and purchase my "Let's Get Better Program" plus paperback books only to be told that because I am not a non-profit person (I tried to be but I'm a conflict of interest lol) that "the vacancy" is no longer available. My camera is still in the pawn shop and I've only sold 4 books to help cover the cost of Business Permit as I will still need one of those.

The Let's Get Better Program is for the town I'm an immigrant in because they are not Bipolar nor tourist friendly. I could write on thousands of postcards without a problem, "Whether you like it or not welcome to the town I   reside   in."

The Difference between Need and Want

I could begin this post with what inspired me to write about the difference between knowing what the difference between needing someone or something versus wanting someone or something but my inspiration shall remain anonymous as per usual. As a person with counseling skills, I found it rather strange at this day and age that one does not understand the difference or if they do know what the difference is that they are misusing it.

Comparison of perceptional needs could be considered as:

One needs to drink water but they may not want to.

One needs to eat food but they may not want to.

One wants help but they may not need it.

One wants to have everything but they may not need it.

One may want to get married but they do not need to.

One needs emotions but they may not want them.

One may need to ask for help but the want to ask is reluctant.

When we acknowledge the difference between the two and how more often than not, we say we need something when really, we just want.

My next favorite is not looking like somebody who needs help but really they do the vice versa how looking like someone who is in need of help and they take it to the "award ceremony" relying on "I need this, I need that, I need a man, I need a child, I need a woman, I need, I need" whereas all of these are just wants. If somebody is truly done they need to learn how to do things themselves or resign themselves to the pity pot existence of thinking that everyone needs to help when nobody wants to.

I like help but I do not require or need it. This statement would be the difference between empowering and in power.

Understanding Repeated Exposure

More often than not society appears to be blissful about what and how repeated exposure is inter-connected to Bipolar Disorder and the mental condition of an individual who experiences any type of constant negative repeated exposure. It could be a sound, a tone, a voice, being put on hold for countless minute which deems the beginning stem of anxieties cause by repeated exposure.

It seems as though there are many perfectly chemically balanced individuals out there or those who deem themselves to have a chemical balance therefore no out bursts of anger, hostility do not occur or maybe they do but they deem themselves to be of a lesser emotional range of a person with a type of Bipolar Disorder.

To try and explain verbally is almost futile. Pre-formed judgement, perception, angst, values of the chemically balanced feels unconquerable as they spout their opinions, thoughts, values, feelings before a person with a type of Bipolar Disorder can fully explain why and the incidences that occurred to be deemed as outrageous behavior of course that is deemed by the ones who are chemically balanced or claim to be of such "value".

One method of trying to release because they deem your behavior outrageous and somehow it is difficult to let go when they aren't listening. Oh sure they are standing in front of you but their ears are closed and those beady black eyes cast their angst. Remind yourself that they are the ones who deem themselves to be of sound mind, body and soul. One method that I think would be highly effective because I'm "willing to go there" is to obtain the release required so this outrageous behavior is discontinued. Important Note: the "individual" needs to be willing to exercise restraint in speaking and a willingness to grasp the metaphor being used. I call it **"The Rock in the Bucket Method"**

It all starts with empty buckets and with your willing individual who is willing to help you move through this mental state. That person is hold the buck and you start at the beginning of the repeated exposure "gone bad". Make sure you find the appropriate size of rock to indicate the "effect" that situation created. Some may need more buckets, some people may need less and congratulations if you don't have very many rocks in your bucket.

As the bucket becomes full, the person has to continue to carry that bucket and when the second bucket is full or when they start to complain about the "weight" of the rocks allow them to use a method of transporting them while you fill up two more buckets until all the incidences are gone or "removed from the memory bank". When your person starts complaining so much you can't take it anymore or they just plain stop you say to them "That is my repeated exposure and what I have been carrying around while you say I am acting outrageously. Oh and please stop complaining because you are chemically balanced and chemically balanced people can take the weight of incidence like this, they are supposed to be light as a feather."

Since I have not been able to perform this method I am unable to show the "value" in which this is understood. What I do have is another example of what it is like for a person with a type of Bipolar Disorder.

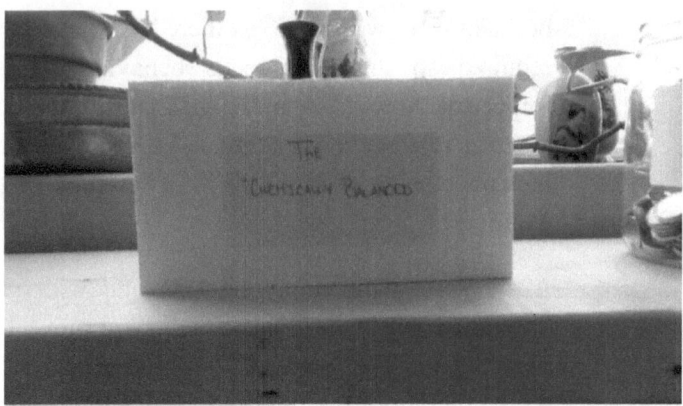

In this photo, it is a representation of a person who is "right as rain". Please note the Styrofoam and how that relates to their behaviors.

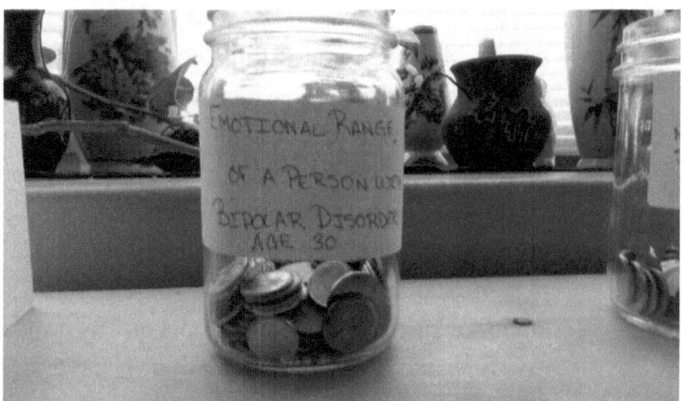

This is a representation of a person who has a type of Bipolar Disorder who typically speaking is beginning the route of taking medication. Please note the pennies, and nickels. They represent the "value" of each incident. This person is starting to take their medication regularly.

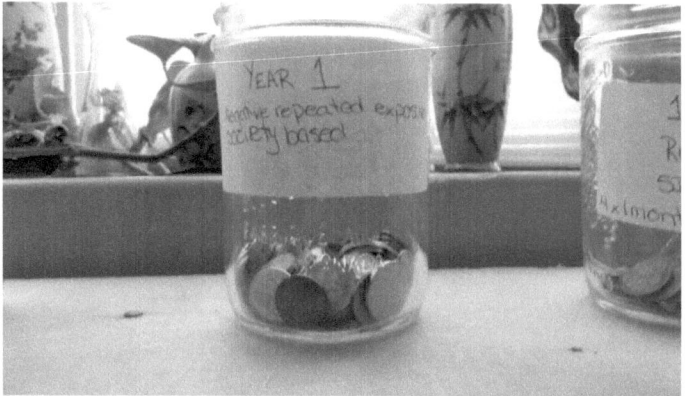

This is a representation of a person with a type of Bipolar Disorder entering into a new situation such as a new job, new town on a society based level.

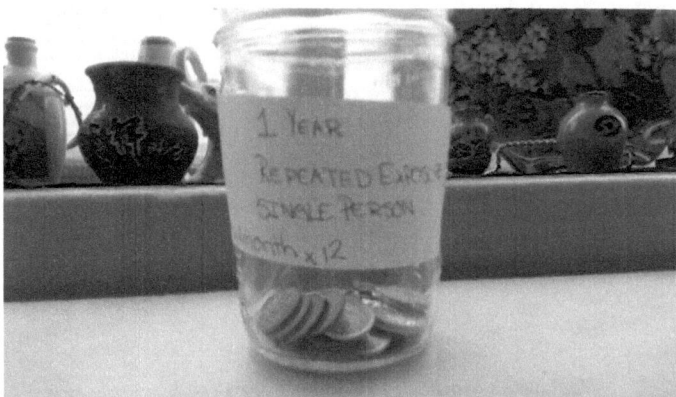

This is a representation of a person with a type of Bipolar Disorder that interacts with an individual on average of 4 times per month multiplied by one year. You will notice that there are some dimes, nickels, and pennies indicating value.

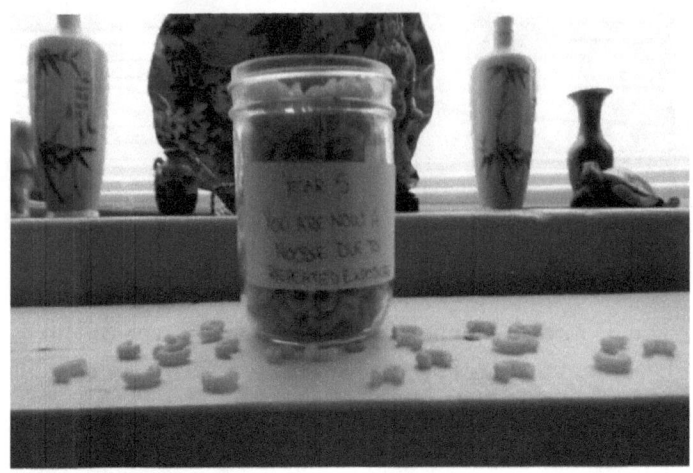

This is a representation of the fifth year of unresolved repeated exposure. Please note that in the photo it is noodles as the representation because this is when you are being told you are acting outrageously. The scattered macaroni indicates that the person has become overwhelmed and this is collateral damage.

Taking the "Bull" Out of Bipolar for the Sake of Hierarchy

One of the most challenging behaviors to keep under control is "THE BULL".

The bull is the one that within five minutes has a thousand ideas and a few more thousand questions of why, and how about this. The bull also is charging up for the task at hand; thinking of ways for perfection, creating new "modules" for the "elders of hierarchy".

The Bull works constantly; it has little or no need for sleep. It wants to go all out and be the Tasmanian Devil but after the whirlwind it's sparkly, and beautiful in the eyes of the now "spent" Bull.

The Bull doesn't work well under rules or having to deal with a whole bunch of people to have the one answer it wants; which of course is "yes". The Bull can run like the wind, snorting, ripping, tearing up the land, and yet it can stand still for several hours' content to watch life go by. When that Bull gets going and it's not like they mean to be of this way; it is in their nature to be so bold, forthright, captivating in the variety of new eyes that sparkle with delight and shades.

There are two sides to the Bull; the one that is positive and the one that is negative.

A negative Bull is the one that has tons of experience yet ends up in a low wage paying job that only uses ten percent of their true capacity. They want to be number one, they want to be in charge, and they will keep making suggestions until you tire of them.

The positive Bull is the one who has the in charge capabilities and despite the inner turmoil accepts that hierarchy is their way. It might be the correct way but as a Bull it is no easy task to just let go of things while the rest of the world does their thing.

We have to remember this is the Bulls' life and precipices come and somehow when leaks occur it falls apart at the last moment even though it was whipped together by a Tasmanian Devil while the world is right as rain.

There is Always One

More often than not there will always be one object, thingymabob, person, food item, piece of clothing, DVD, collectible antique, one train of thought, and there always is one that talks on and on about everything under the sun even the simplest of things to be looked upon in a way that one never thought about before.

It seems as though I have stories that start out with, "This one time...." As there is always room for one more story of laugher and how the perceptional view of others is often tainted by preformed ideas of "what is good and what is not." There is always one of my non-emotionally supportive persons in my life who likes to say, "Get a job." I usually reply "Yes" as I explore another medium of artistry that is no Mona Lisa but I am just what is termed as "playing" and I should be selling instead of giving because with wisdom it would be unwise to playful art beside majestic art.

I realize that I live in a very odd area to be "emerging" from but welcome to not having the ability to change locations to associate the "proper perceptions of a person to be 'good or bad' or to be deemed another 'craazzeee'". Now I am probably judged as being crazy and I accept that because as a person with a type of Bipolar Disorder who has read several self-help books, attended counseling, written two self-help books about Bipolar Disorder and have attempted to end the physical body presence so that the "most important part" can be moved to a better location. Wouldn't that be nice? To say, "Give me a different one, this one isn't working properly and why do I always get the wrong one?"

There will always be one that objects to such thoughts that the One has quite the sense of humor "using" his gifted as yo yo's and likes to provide the most challenges as there will always be one more to go and just when you think there will be no more there is another one around the corner. Oh and how there is always one more lesson to be learned.

To be deemed, "there is always one" in a media field, in my perception the one would be signing up for GoggleBox, write on Facebook professional fan pages, do a Twitter shout-out every day to my favorite reality TV shows which are mostly gold mining. Another "there is always one" is writing on Facebook every day how much I love my favorite reality TV persons and whom I do not deem worthy of being a boss and of course I always use humor. I consider myself to be a "couch mining expert" as there is always one of those LOL! Truthfully being a couch mining expert I have watched 14 different mining operations and most of the segments show how to fix something and mining techniques that are successful and some, well, I think that they put those people on there just for poking fun at. It does seem like there is always one of those.

This one time, actually as of late I am finding that there is always one time during a moment in the day that negative words are spewed out in a less than worthy way. Every situation there is always one out-burst of negativity, there is no making fun of the situation, or being agreeable to what is happening as it isn't as "good as" one wants it. There will always be one time or another that all of it becomes too much. More so for the one that learned one has to be happy all the time or another that all of it becomes too much. More so for the one that learned one has to be happy all the time in order to maintain the happy endorphin's because there will always be one time or another that happiness is required to compensate for the level of irritated "ness" of the one who is always the one to freak out; throw things, or curse excessively.

As I take out my frustration in painting because there is always one who seems to think that I'm a "fruitcake" or "who would do that? Oh yeah, she's one of those." Now unfortunately I am not famous or "noteworthy" enough to have reprints or the ability to redo things exactly the same as the last time. Also there is always one that pokes fun at persons who regard art found in reprints.

I am also "always the one" to give my work always as I have great difficulty pricing my "exploring playful fun" because if I price it too high I'm considered always the one to be "out to lunch" on pricing and if I price too low I'd be considered to be "always the one" that does not consider my work to be worthy of large denominational selling price.

If you can't see the photos there is always one that doesn't seem work and a conspiracy theory evolves and well there is always one who doesn't believe in freedom of speech and there is always one that doesn't respect others and their "standing in life due to geographical location".

More Often Than Not

Do you ever find that during the day you have a list of things that need to be done but more often than not they are never completed?

It's typical that more often than not our wants or needs get dismissed by what could be determined as the regularly scheduled routine. As a person with a type of Bipolar Disorder more often than not I find myself waiting to do things and when the time finally comes, more often than not become deflated and it is not completed or started.

Typically speaking, persons with a type of Bipolar Disorder prefer consistency because it helps create a continuous flow of upward movement. More often than not, this doesn't happen as often as one would hope. Learning to deal with a constant cycle of change can be quite difficult. As an example; every two weeks it rotates between the ability to accomplish tasks during the day or trying to accomplish tasks in the afternoon and into the evening.

The first tell-tale sign of a change taking place would be in the kitchen because maybe it's Monday and you just spent the weekend enjoying activities and the dishes aren't done up to date. Another sign is laundry; more often than not the clothes take a journey from the floor to the washing machine to the dryer then in a laundry hamper where it stays or until it's gone through looking for clean clothes. (Who said one needed a dresser anyways? Lol just kidding). Another sign would be the lack of dirty dishes in the sink when it's the afternoon/evening cycle.

So many times we begin to start and the eyes become shiny with passion then interrupted by reality because more often than not we wake up too early, make too much noise, are considered lazy, it's not time yet, and finally where did the day go? More often than not another day passes and it's the same as the day before. A good more often than not is finding yourself wanting to do something but you have to get dressed, do your hair, etc etc and the important thing you were eager to do well, more often than not the lack of drive by the afternoon makes for a better snooze than a productive time.

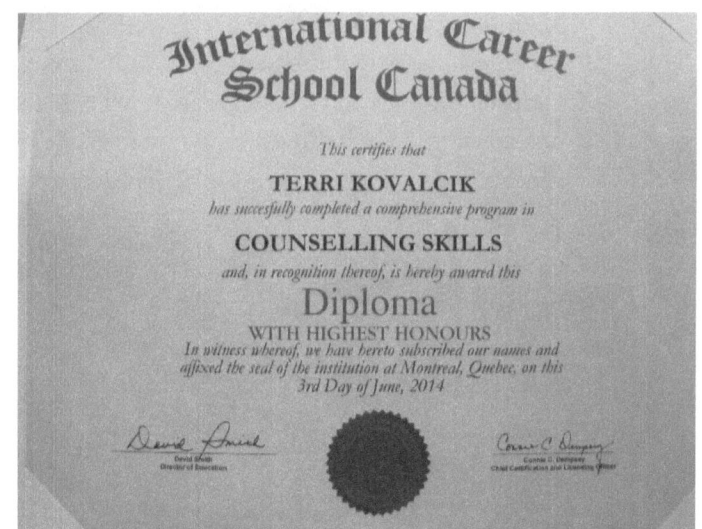

Terri Kovalciks'

Top 4 Social Media Sites

www.tlctouchedwithfire.wordpress.com

www.facebook.com/tlctouchedwithfire

www.facebook.com/JuniorHuntersatLarge

www.facebook.com/TheBipolarWorkshop

.

Other Titles Available

By Terri Kovalcik

- Junior Hunters at Large Series;
  - Volume 1 A Year of Sportsmanship
  - Volume 2 Year of the Sportsman
- The Bipolar Workshop
- I Was So Bipolar
- Sparkly, The Pink Unicorn; In the Land of Rainbows
- The Dare
- Funny Short Stories For Kids
- Hunting and Fishing For Kids
- Mortal Love
- Let's Make A Book
- Close Encounters of the Bipolar Mind
- Revelance; A Time Period
- Scripts: Glorification Series:
  - Lest We Forget Jonah
  - After and Among Us
  - Old Words New

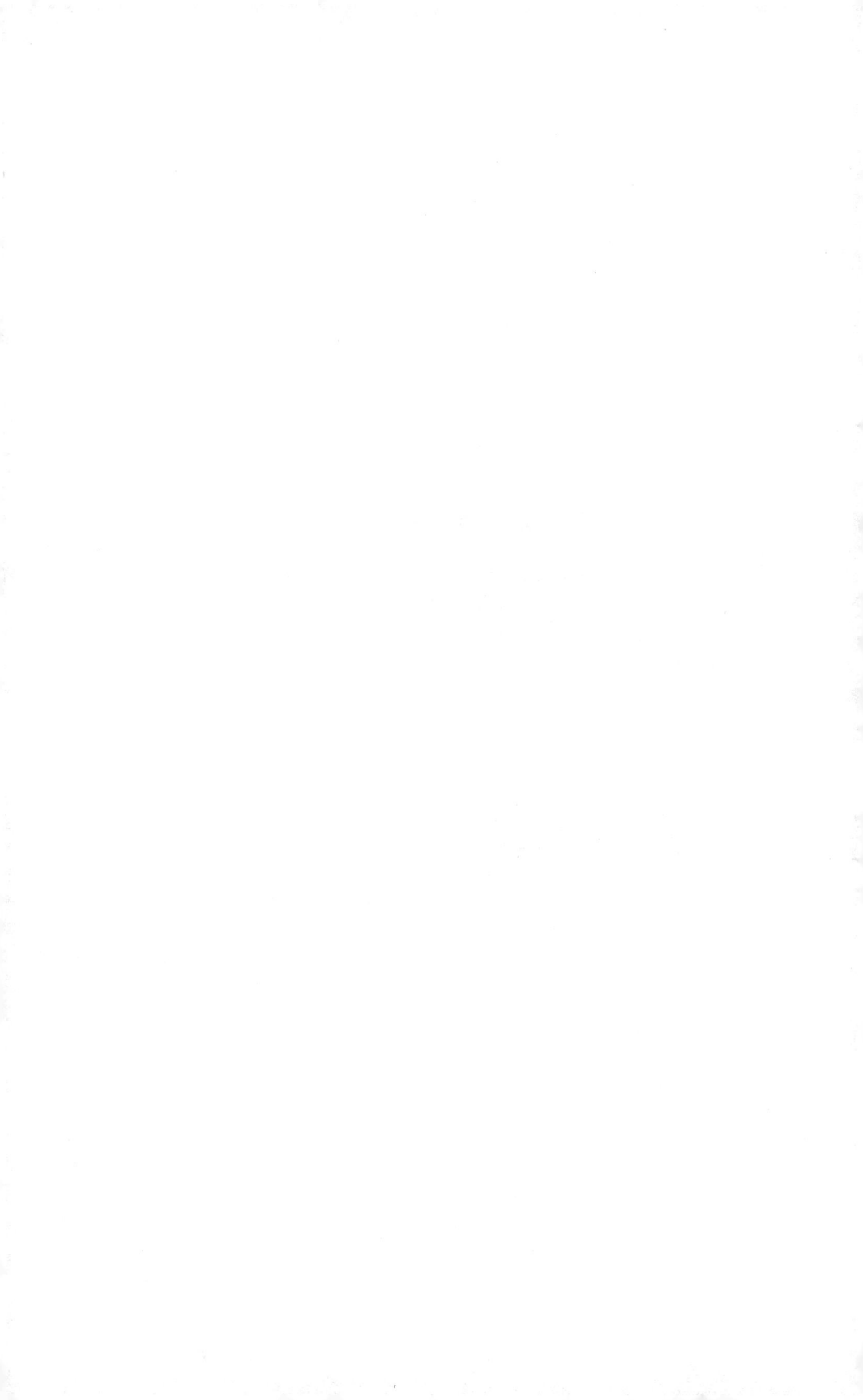